THE EASY NO-FLAB DIET

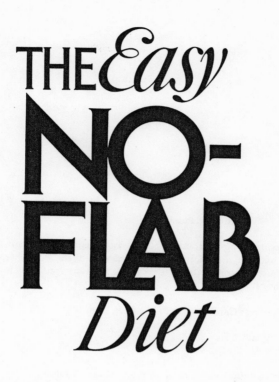

THE *Easy* NO-FLAB *Diet*

RICHARD PASSWATER

RICHARD MAREK PUBLISHERS
NEW YORK

Library of Congress Cataloging in Publication Data

Passwater, Richard A
  The easy no-flab diet.

  1. Reducing diets.   2. Food—Composition—Tables.
I. Title.
RM222.2.P35   613.2'5   79-4684
ISBN 0-399-90034-9

Printed in the United States of America

Fourth Impression

To my mother, not only because she awakened my interest in nutrition when I was ten by giving me Victor Lindlahr's book, *You Are What You Eat,* but for all those loving things that mothers do for their children and for which they rarely receive thanks.

Mabel K. Passwater of Wilmington, Delaware.

ACKNOWLEDGEMENTS

Aside from the many research reports that the Easy No-Flab Diet is based on, many people have helped me with their ideas and time. I offer them special thanks.

Foremost I owe thanks to Diane Raintree for convincing me to omit many boring technical explanations, and editing my scientific writing toward a modern fluent style.

My wife, Barbara, deserves special praise for helping me meet deadlines by sacrificing her time to pitch in with the typing and for her skillful critiques.

The contributions of the following people are deeply appreciated: Rheo Blair, Herb Boynton, Dr. Richard O. Brennan, Dr. Keith Brewer, Dr. Ray Chen, Joe Coffini, Dr. Carlton Fredericks, Jerry Gillman, Wayne Harris, Don Heidi, Dr. James Julian, Mort Katz, Dr. Hans Kugler, Dr. Steve Langer, Dr. Carl Miller, Dr. Dave Miller, Robert Orben, Lou Rinaldi, Irv Rosenberg, R.Ph., Ron Sell, Allen Skolnick, Harald Taub, Anthony Umbdenstock, Larry Westfall, and Dr. Roger Williams.

CONTENTS

FOREWORD

AS A PHYSICIAN WHO HAS TREATED more than 50,000 obese patients, I am dubious of the appearance of another diet book. Nevertheless I read every one of them in the hope of finding basic, useful information.

Unfortunately, the more of these books overweight people read, the more confused they are likely to become. My patients have often asked why someone can't come up with an easy system that works, and doesn't require the calculations and planning of a computer technician. I have often wondered the same thing and wished I could devise such a method.

Now, it has been done! I breathe a sigh of relief with my patients and join them in celebrating this accomplishment by Richard Passwater, which might result in their liberation from confusion and discouragement.

The Easy No-Flab Diet represents a dramatic new approach to weight-loss. I foresee the extensive use of this book as a reference work for physicians as well as patients and its use as a manual for serious weight watchers.

11

Conscientious use of this book could well make any other "how to diet" book unnecessary.

JAMES J. JULIAN, M.D.
Hollywood, California.

PREFACE

HOW MANY TIMES HAVE YOU SAID "I hardly eat a thing and I can't lose a pound"? I said that a number of times myself until I learned that many fat people eat less than most thin people do. It's just that they have a fat person's body chemistry and they don't know what to do about it.

I have been helping people reduce and build muscle on a professional basis since 1960, first as a spa instructor and then as a research consultant and nutritional advisor for an international weight-loss guidance firm. During that time I've seen many popular diets come and go.

Why was I, as a biochemist, interested in helping people lose weight? It was an opportunity for me to have unlimited use of one of the finest health spas in order to continue body-building with weights and exercise apparatus.

During the previous three years I had put on 60 pounds of muscle, and during the first 2 years as a spa instructor I gained another 20 pounds of muscle.

Then I got married, opened my own lab, wrote technical reference books, and stopped heavy weight-training. I no longer burned thousands of calories in heavy exercise,

13

but much of my appetite remained. The muscle was replaced by flab.

Fortunately, the change didn't occur overnight, and I've had the opportunity to experiment with reducing diets as I lost 50 pounds of flab. That's when I really learned the difference between weight-loss and fat-loss. Any reducing diet produces weight-loss, but dieters really want to lose fat.

My first-hand experience in paring off flab, my own and that of the hundreds of people I helped at the spa, was a good foundation for me when I became a research consultant and nutritional advisor for an international weight-loss corporation.

Through a North American and European network of weight-loss counselors, I was able to expand my involvement with reducing diets and their problems to over 200,000 successful dieters. It is reasonable to say that before developing the Easy No-Flab Diet, I was associated with dieters losing over 1,000 tons of body fat.

Recent findings from dozens of biochemistry, nutrition, and sports medicine laboratories are the basis of the Easy No-Flab Diet.

My major contribution is the development of the FLAB Unit concept and the FLAB Index. I hope they prove useful for dieters who have tried to be naturally slender and found it wasn't easy, and for those who have never needed to diet and want to keep it that way.

The Easy No-Flab Diet has been favorably reviewed by several qualified experts in universities and federal agencies concerned with health and nutrition. It has been found successful by the Total Woman Spas headquartered in San Diego, California.

It works and it is safe. I urge you to give it a try. You'll be glad you did!

IT'S NOT WEIGHT
YOU WANT TO LOSE,
BUT FAT

1 TRIMMING YOUR WAISTLINE DOESN'T
have to be complicated or frustrating. The good
news is that you can become naturally slender
while enjoying delicious foods. You don't have to go hungry. You don't have to worry about calories. You don't
have to have strong willpower. The Easy No-Flab Diet
will liberate pounds of fat tissue without complication or
frustration. And it will improve your health, figure, and
skin.

I mention *fat* tissue because most dieters think in
terms of *weight* loss. Much of the weight lost on low-carbohydrate diets, "crash diets," or other "fad" diets is essential lean tissue. That's not the weight dieters should
be losing. It's fat tissue they should be shedding, and the
Easy No-Flab Diet will help them do just that. It's possible to lose "inches" of flab without actual weight loss.
Muscle tissue is more dense, thus an equal weight of
muscle occupies less space. You can build your figure
with exercise at the same time you burn flab.

Close to 10 million adults are actually on one reducing
diet or another as you read this chapter. Because many of
these dieters have chosen a less-than-perfect diet, they

15

may be doomed to riding a "roller coaster" of weight-loss/weight-gain for the rest of their lives.

There are many "diets" around that will help you lose pounds—but most help you lose more than fat. You can lose weight on a cookie diet or a carrot diet, but you could also lose your hair, your resistance to infection, your "sanity," or your life.

Nearly all reducing diets will help you lose weight if you follow them. But most dieters find that the common-sense, low-calorie diets leave them too hungry to stick with it long enough to lose appreciable weight. Or they find that the crash diets don't train them to eat nutritionally when the diet is over. Thus, they gain weight while the roller-coaster effect of weight-loss and weight-gain continues. And fad diets are downright dangerous!

The point is to lose not only weight, or pounds, but also to lose *flab* without losing needed lean tissue and energy, or putting the body through stress.

Losing fat is more involved than simply losing weight. Factors such as food quantity, food quality, the timing of meals, the severity of the calorie reduction, and the rate of weight-loss must be controlled in order to safely lose flab without losing needed tissue.

The Easy No-Flab Diet controls each of these factors for you. The result is that the weight you lose comes from your fat cells, not from the cells of your muscles or vital organs—as is the dangerous result of crash or fad diets. Yet you will lose pounds of fat rapidly without hunger.

If you are more than 20 pounds overweight, you can expect to lose 13 to 30 pounds of *fat* a month, while those with less to lose will lose their fat proportionately slower.

Even the differences between men and women in hormonal activity and the number of fat cells are taken into account in the Easy No-Flab Diet. It's more difficult for women to lose fat, so they are given special help.

And speaking of help, you will learn a quick trick to stop hunger by finger pressure on a spot near your ear. It's sort of an acupuncture-without-needles technique. And, like the Easy No-Flab Diet, it works.

DON'T COUNT CALORIES—
COUNT FLABS

2 THE EASY NO-FLAB DIET IS BASED ON A principle that has been understood for some time. The principle is that proper control of the blood-sugar level prevents hunger and controls the burning of body fat.

The factor of key importance in controlling the blood-sugar level is the rate at which the hormone insulin is released from the pancreas. And it's food quality that determines this rate of insulin release, as much as it's how much and how often you eat.

The Easy No-Flab Diet controls insulin release as well as how much and how often you eat, so that you lose fat at the maximum safe rate. Believe it or not, eating several small meals a day melts fat away much more quickly than eating one or two larger meals—even when the total calories are the same in both cases.

GOOD PROTEINS—BAD PROTEINS

The Easy No-Flab Diet Program doesn't simply count calories or grams of carbohydrates or protein but controls the quality of each food in the diet, so that you will lose fat as fast as safely possible. All you have to do is select meals from the many tasty Easy No-Flab Diet Menus. When you want to design your own meals, at any point during the diet, simply turn to the FLAB Index in Appendix III at the back of this book. It will tell you at a glance the number of FLAB units in a standard serving of various foods. You can eat a generous portion of virtually any meat, fish, fowl, vegetable, or fruit, plus a moderate portion of bread, pasta or potatoes at both lunch and dinner. You can enjoy every meal on the Easy No-Flab Diet.

Food quality is important in getting and staying slender. The quality of food is determined by the types of protein and carbohydrate in the food, and by their balance.

There are good proteins and bad proteins. It's the balance of essential amino acids that determines the quality of a protein. Since most whole foods consist of numerous proteins of varying quality, there is a need for a convenient index of food quality. The FLAB Index created especially for this book meets that need for dieters.

There are good carbohydrates and bad carbohydrates. It all depends on whether they maintain or disrupt the blood-sugar level. Most foods consist of several types of carbohydrates, but until the development of the FLAB Index, foods have not been quality-rated with the dieter in mind.

Fortunately, food quality, in terms of controlling body fat, can now be easily determined by simply turning to the FLAB Index. The special feature of this index is that it offers a unit of measurement far more reliable than the calorie unit for predicting the gaining or losing of fat—the FLAB Unit.

THE FLAB UNIT

The term FLAB stands for Fat Liquidating Ability Barometer. Figure 2-1 shows two FLAB Barometers illustrating the difference in the Fat Liquidating Ability of a hamburger and a jelly donut. Although the hamburger and the jelly donut both contain 250 calories, the donut has twice as many FLAB Units and would be a poor selection in a diet aimed at burning body fat.

The calorie unit, a measure not relied on in the Easy No-Flab Diet, reflects only the potential energy of the food and does not tell us much about anything else. One calorie unit may come from a simple carbohydrate, such as table sugar, or from a complex carbohydrate such as those in whole grains or fibrous vegetables, or even from protein or fat.

The catch is that the body doesn't handle food in terms of calories. It handles food in terms of protein quality, carbohydrate quality, and fat quality. Science uses the calorie unit to measure all types of energy, for our convenience in understanding various processes. But, if we limit food description to energy concepts, we lose sight of

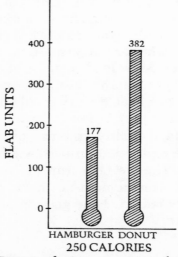

Figure 2-1 Donut calories are twice as fattening as hamburger's. Compare the FLAB Units in 250 calories of donuts (two plain cake-type donuts or one jelly donut) with the FLAB Units in 250 calories of hamburger (4 oz).

20

TABLE 2-1

Food	Quantity	Prote (g)	Carbo (g)	Fat (g)	Cals	FLABs
Donut (cake-type)	2	2.5	33	12	250	382
Hamburger	4 oz	31	0	12.8	248	177

the actual processes that are occurring because each type of calorie is handled differently by the body. And not surprisingly, each type of calorie has a separate influence on fat storage. The general rule is that *empty* calorie foods make *full* pounds of body fat!

The calorie unit is not a good one to rely on if you want to lose flab and stay naturally slender. But you can rely on the FLAB Unit. One FLAB Unit of a simple carbohydrate will have the same fat-storing ability as one FLAB Unit of protein.

The FLAB Index listing the FLAB Units for all the foods most frequently eaten is given in Appendix III. Table 2-1 indicates the FLAB Units in just two of the foods listed in the FLAB Index. You don't have to worry about the number of FLAB Units in the food you eat on the Easy No-Flab Diet when you rely on the suggested menus for your meals. If you want to create your own meals at any point during the diet, the FLAB Index will provide an easy guide to designing meals that will keep you losing flab until you are naturally slender.

Let's look at some examples to illustrate the difference between counting calories and counting FLABs. One jelly-filled donut or two small cake-type donuts contain 250 calories, the same number as a 4-oz hamburger patty. However, the hamburger contains only 177 FLABs, while there are 382 FLABs in the two cake-type donuts or one jelly-filled donut. Although the calorie count is the same, the donuts are more than twice as fattening as the hamburger. The FLAB Barometers shown in Figure 2-1 help illustrate the difference. Table 2-1 shows where that difference comes from. The donut contains more FLAB Units because of its large number of grams of simple carbohydrates, which produce more fat.

Let's compare eggs and ice cream. One-half pint (1 cup) of vanilla ice cream contains 275 calories, the same as 3⅓ hard-boiled eggs. Yet the ice cream is more than 1⅔ times as fattening. See Figure 2-2 and Table 2-2 for illustrations of the reasons why.

Do you want another example? Compare a milk chocolate bar of about an ounce to three slices of Swiss cheese. Both contain about 150 calories, but the candy bar is 1⅔ times as fattening as the cheese. See Figure 2-3 and Table 2-3.

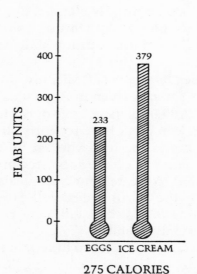

275 CALORIES

Figure 2-2 Ice cream is more than 1⅔ times as fattening as eggs. Compare the FLAB Units in 275 calories of ice cream (1 cup) with the FLAB Units in 275 calories of eggs (3⅓ hard-boiled).

22

TABLE 2-2–2-3

Food	Quantity	Prote (g)	Carbo (g)	Fat (g)	Cals	FLABs
Eggs	3.3 large	21.6	1.6	19.3	273	223
Ice cream	1 cup	5.4	27.4	16.6	276	379
Swiss cheese	3 slices	12.0	0.7	11.6	154	131
Choco-late bar	1 oz	2.2	16.1	9.2	147	219

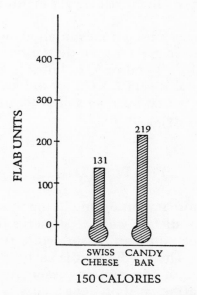

Figure 2-3 A chocolate candy bar is 1⅔ times as fattening as 3 slices of Swiss cheese. Compare the FLAB Units in 150 calories of the candy bar (1 oz) with the FLAB Units in 150 calories (3 slices) of Swiss cheese.

23

There you have just three examples of the differences between FLAB Units and calorie units.

THE FLAB CONCEPT

The body handles sugars (simple carbohydrates) and starches (complex carbohydrates) in different ways; and it handles proteins and fats still differently.

It's not only how much potential energy is in the food that counts in losing flab and maintaining energy, but how fast the food digests, how concentrated the carbohydrates are, how balanced the amino acids are, and even something called nutrient density. All these factors determine whether a food will trigger fat storage or satisfy hunger.

The differences among foods in allowing stored fat to be burned are even greater than their differences in making fat. Basically all you need to know is that the FLAB Index assigns values (FLAB Units) to food according to the fat-storing and fat-burning ability (or insulin-release-stimulating ability) of the food.

THE FLAB INDEX

Fat-loss is more important in dieting than weight-loss. In other words, dieters want to preserve (that is, spare) their needed lean (protein) tissue while trimming away their fat tissue. The FLAB Index is useful here because it is an indicator of the protein-preserving and insulin-release-stimulating capability of a food.

A food that preserves lean tissue perfectly or does not cause a *flood* of insulin to flow into the bloodstream is rated as 100.0. The lower the rating on the FLAB Index,

24

the less suitable a food is for trimming away fat preferentially.

Tuna, ham and T-bone steak are excellent protein-preserving foods and have FLAB Indexes of 93.0, 91.7, and 90.0, respectively. Poor-quality foods such as a sugar cookie, devil's food cake and table sugar have FLAB Indexes of 38.6, 35.6, and 31.0 respectively.

Any food having a FLAB Index less than 50 should be avoided during a fat-loss diet and eaten only on rare occasions by successful ex-dieters and those who have never needed to diet.

Table 2-4 lists the FLAB Index for several frequently eaten foods. Before you start the Easy No-Flab Diet, you'll want to turn to Appendix III. It lists the FLAB Index for essentially all of the frequently eaten foods.

Figure 2-4 illustrates the factors that determine the FLAB rating of a food. (A simple guide to FLAB rating can be approximated by assigning a gram of sugar twice the number of FLAB Units as a gram of complex carbohy-

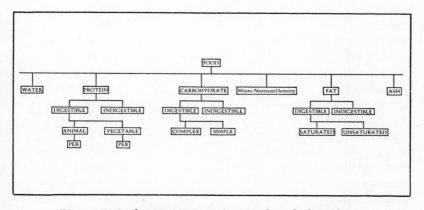

Figure 2-4 The FLAB Concept. A detailed analysis of food subclasses helps explain a food's ability to contribute to the fat-burning or fat-storing metabolism.

TABLE 2-4
Sample Listing of FLAB Index

This list has been selected to illustrate the range of food quality available. The keystone of any diet should be foods with a high FLAB Index (above 75). Foods having a FLAB Index above 50 can be used to balance the meals nutritionally and add flavor and variety to mealtimes. Foods having a FLAB Index below 50 should be eaten only occasionally—never when dieting. (The FLAB Index is obtained by multiplying the number of calories in a portion by 62 and then dividing by the number of FLAB Units in that portion.)

Foods	FLAB Index
Broiled fish	100.0
Veal	99.7
Roasted chicken	97.9
Tuna	93.0
Ham	91.7
T-Bone steak	90.0
Fried chicken	87.8
Cottage cheese	84.5
Liver	84.0
Corn, an ear	81.2
Skim milk	77.0
Breaded fish	76.8
Boiled egg	75.9
Carrot, cooked	75.8
Mashed potato	72.8
Yogurt, strawberry	67.7
Whole wheat bread	66.9
Peas, green	64.4
Banana	63.7
Orange juice	63.1
Grapefruit	62.0
Ice Cream, vanilla	45.0
Jelly	41.1
Sugar cookie	38.6
Pie, apple	38.6

Food	FLAB Index
Cake, sponge	36.3
Cake, devil's food	35.6
Candy Bar, milk chocolate	32.2
Soda, cola	31.2
Sugar	31.0

drate, and by assigning a gram of poor-quality protein 50 percent more FLAB Units than high-quality protein.) It may sound like a math problem, but relax—you don't have to do the math. The Easy No-Flab Index has done it for you. The "FLAB" principles of FLAB Units and FLAB Index have been published for scientific review in *Nutritional Perspectives* (Vol 2 #1, pp. 32–45, January 1979).

NUTRIENT DENSITY

The FLAB Index considers only the effect of the food on controlling body fat and is not a measure of vitamin and mineral quality. The term for the measure of vitamin and mineral quality is "nutrient density." Nutrient density is considered in the formulation of the FLAB Index and FLAB Units, but need not be considered here. You can trust the fact that all foods in the Easy No-Flab Diet are relatively high in nutrient density.

THE EASY NO-FLAB DIET MEAL

It's foods that have a high rank in the FLAB Index that comprise every meal in the Easy No-Flab Diet.

Because moderate amounts of carbohydrates are part of the diet, the serious problems of the low-carbohydrate,

TABLE 2–5
High-Quality Foods

The following foods have been selected from each major food group as examples of high-quality foods. Just a few of the foods from each group are presented as a sample of the FLAB Index.

Food Group	FLAB Index
Milk	
Cottage cheese	84.5
Buttermilk	79.1
Skim milk	77.0
Swiss cheese	73.4
Whole milk	68.6
Meat	
Broiled fish	100.0
Veal	99.7
Roasted chicken	97.9
Roasted turkey	94.8
Roasted beef, ground	86.7
Fruit	
Apples	69.9
Prunes	68.3
Oranges	66.1
Apricots	65.4
Strawberries	62.0
Vegetable	
Cabbage	100.0
Carrots (raw)	100.0
Celery	100.0
Lettuce	100.0
Grains	
Corn flakes	72.0
Tortilla	69.8
Whole wheat bread	66.9
Pancakes	64.1
Spaghetti	63.6

Food	FLAB Index
Combinations	
Chicken Salad Sandwich	77.9
Roast Beef Sandwich	77.8
Tunafish Salad Sandwich	74.9
Snacks	
Popcorn, plain	100.0
Peanuts,	
dry roasted	72.3
Gelatin, dietetic	
(unsweetened)	70.9
Apple	69.9
Cereal, puffed	
(unsweetened)	68.0
Pickles	64.0

high-protein diets—hunger, irritability, loss of energy, nausea, diarrhea, insomnia and vomiting—are avoided. Complex carbohydrates, such as the starches in potatoes, pastas, and breads, enter the bloodstream evenly over a long period of time and do not disrupt the hunger and fat-burning controls, as do sugars. That's why including appropriate amounts of them in the diet will not slow down a dieter's fat-loss.

Sugars, especially refined sugars, digest rapidly and enter the bloodstream as a concentrated shot, which disrupts the hunger and fat-burning controls. That's why everyone—non-dieters included—should avoid them.

A meal consisting of nearly a quarter pound of protein plus a quarter pound of complex carbohydrates, with little simple carbohydrate and virtually no refined sugar, is perfect for safely controlling body fat. Each meal on the Easy No-Flab Diet is just that.

All you have to do to keep from setting off your hunger

and fat-storage triggers is to eat meals before your periods of greatest activity and avoid foods that trip these triggers.

Your meals should be relatively larger earlier in the day and lighter at dinner than you are currently accustomed to. As an old German adage advises: Breakfast like a king, lunch like a prince, and dine like a pauper. And you'll be naturally slender, as you want to be.

ADVANTAGES OF THE
EASY NO-FLAB DIET

3 TRADITIONAL DIETS DO NOT TAKE AD-vantage of the different effects that proteins, fats, and carbohydrates have in burning stored body fat or in eliminating pangs of hunger. Low-calorie diets merely stress calorie reduction. Unfortunately, much of the weight lost by people on low-calorie diets may be essential lean tissue.

DISADVANTAGES OF LOW-CALORIE DIETS

Low-calorie diets limit essential nutrients as well as calories. But the biggest disadvantage for dieters is that low-calorie diets cause such gyrations in the hunger-control system that few people have the tremendous will-power required to withstand the hunger caused by the diets long enough to lose appreciable weight. Dr. George Blackburn, of the Center for Nutritional Research in Boston, finds that only one in twenty people can stay on a standard low-calorie diet for twelve weeks or more. And only one in twenty can actually lose more than 40 pounds. The temptation to cheat is always there because of gnawing hunger.

DISADVANTAGES OF LOW-CARBOHYDRATE DIETS

The newer low-carbohydrate diets leave many people fatigued, weak, irritable, depressed, and nervous. Unfortunately, much of the weight lost by people on low-carbohydrate diets may be essential lean tissue or simply water loss due to their diuretic action. Once a normal amount of carbohydrate returns to the diet, the weight returns as the body returns to normal fluid levels. The devastating weight rebound usually carries the dieter to an even higher weight. Dr. James Julian, the famous diet specialist of Hollywood, helped pioneer low-carbohydrate diets 20 years ago, and points out that they should only be used for short periods and under the care of medical specialists. No such problems are created by the Easy No-Flab Diet. The reason is that the No-Flab Diet preferentially burns away body fat rather than body protein while controlling hunger.

While on the diet, and after you've lost all the weight you want to, you will be provided with the greatest amount of nutrients per calorie of food. You will cheerfully lose fat without starvation or fasts, hunger pangs or drugs, shots or artificial sweeteners. The Easy No-Flab diet tastes delicious, has hunger-satisfying bulk, and many taste variations. It's the natural path to safe and effective fat-loss.

PROVE IT YOURSELF

The next time you're hungry try eating 250 calories of a sugary processed food. When hunger strikes again, eat 250 calories of natural food. Compare the length of the times before you were hungry again. One time you might eat a jelly donut, 250 calories of mostly simple carbohydrates; the next time you might eat a hamburger patty, 250 calories of mostly protein. You'll be hungry sooner after eating the jelly donut. Neither snack was a balanced meal, but the hamburger does have more nutrient value than the donut, and it is far better for dieters. The Easy No-Flab Diet is high in hunger-controlling natural foods.

"QUICK" ENERGY FOODS USUALLY TURN TO FLAB

The refined carbohydrates in the donut start digesting in the mouth, and rapidly get into the blood as one potent shot of sugar to disrupt blood-sugar control. The initial burst of blood sugar will provide a shot of "quick" energy for a few minutes, but since the body can't burn that much sugar that quickly, the body's blood-sugar control system is brought into play to prevent the continued rise of this potentially dangerous excess sugar that could otherwise result in coma. The way this system works may surprise you. The bloodstream gets rid of this dangerous excess sugar by converting it into fat! The fat is actually stored energy. It can be used later *if* the blood-sugar level dips too low. Usually most of it isn't used. People prefer to eat again instead. That's why fat people stay fat. Empty calories produce full pounds.

STARCHY FOODS PRODUCE ENERGY— NOT FLAB

Proteins, fats, and complex carbohydrates, such as the starches in potatoes and bread, digest slowly and trickle into the bloodstream at a rate consistent with optimal blood-sugar level. If optimal amounts of such foods are eaten, the result is decreased hunger and fat. And the constant supply of energy these foods supply makes eating those sugary flab-producing snacks unnecessary.

The potential energy difference between refined carbohydrates and complex carbohydrates is much like the potential heat difference between wood and coal. A wood fire, like refined sugar, burns hot for a short time and dies out, while a coal fire, like complex carbohydrates, never reaches that peak of intense heat, but burns longer, supplying all the heat you need. The Easy No-Flab Diet has plenty of "continuous" energy foods.

THE PROBLEM OF ADDICTION TO SUGARY FOODS

Most overweight people have become addicted to poor-quality fattening foods and find it difficult to stop relying on them. As long as there is as little as 5 percent of these poor-quality foods in the diet, most people will still have a "sweet tooth," and will nearly always feel hungry.

The Easy No-Flab Diet quickly breaks the addiction to sugar and other poor-quality foods without stress, because it adjusts the body chemistry to eliminate the craving.

GTF, A NEW NUTRIENT

Glucose Tolerance Factor (GTF) is a recently discovered nutrient that helps regulate the blood-sugar level without increasing the flow of insulin, which would stop fat-burning. The body can either make GTF or obtain it from food. Many people lose their ability to make their own GTF, probably as a result of the repeated floodings of insulin caused by poor-quality foods. Such people tend to make greater amounts of fat and/or develop diabetes.

The role of GTF is to moderate insulin activity. First

by potentiating the circulating insulin and then, if that is still inadequate, by reducing the amount of fresh insulin required to be released. Thus, the roller-coaster effect on blood sugar is moderated.

Dr. Walter Mertz, chairman of the U.S. Department of Agriculture's Nutrition Institute, is a pioneer in GTF research. Dr. Mertz is trying to identify the factor precisely, and at this time has not established the chemical structure of GTF, only the fact that it consists of the mineral chromium, the vitamin niacin, and a specific combination of amino acids (building blocks of protein). GTF has been found in liver, cheese, whole wheat bread (but not white bread, which contains only one tenth the chromium of whole wheat bread), in beef, brewer's yeast, mushrooms, and black pepper. The quality foods in the Easy No-Flab Diet are rich in GTF.

ADDITIONAL ADVANTAGES OF THE NO-FLAB DIET

The improved body chemistry resulting from the Easy No-Flab Diet will reduce migraine headaches and premenstrual tension. Nor will you have to experience the lightheadedness and weakness common for the first one to three weeks on many low-carbohydrate diets.

The Easy No-Flab Diet is effective because it removes not body protein but flab—even those hard-to-lose last 5 pounds. It works because the chemistry is right.

EASY NO-FLAB DIET
AVOIDS COMMON PROBLEMS

4 THE FIRST QUESTION A POTENTIAL DIET-
er asks about a diet is often, "How fast can I
lose weight?" Everyone who's overweight
wants to go to bed fat and wake up skinny. It might be
nice to lose 10 years of fat accumulation overnight, but a
"crash" weight-loss guarantees you will soon become fat
again. You'll take off and put on 10 pounds over and over
again. Some physicians believe this is worse than leaving
the pounds on in the first place.

Rapid weight-loss and -gain creates stress on the body.
When you take off pounds, your kidneys and liver have to
do extra work. When you put weight on, the blood levels
of fats (mostly triglycerides and cholesterol) increase and
red blood cells stick together to reduce the ability of the
blood to carry oxygen to the cells. That puts stress on the
heart which could lead to heart attack.

Each cycle produces a little less weight-loss and a little
more weight-gain. The object of dieting is to lose fat, but
it is equally important to learn by daily practice how to
keep the fat off.

If you are more than 20 pounds overweight, you can expect to lose more than 13 to 30 pounds of *fat* tissue each

month on the Easy No-Flab Diet. That's more than three pounds of flab each week.

If you have less than 20 pounds to lose, the rate of fat-loss will slacken proportionally, but you can count on losing at least 2 pounds of fat per week until you're down to those last 5 pounds.

Those last 5 pounds are the hardest to lose on a permanent basis, and you can expect to lose them at the rate of about 1 pound per week.

WILL THE WEIGHT I LOSE STAY OFF?

The weight you lose on the No-Flab Diet will stay off because you'll be eating similar foods after the diet—the only difference is you'll be eating more of them. The ultimate success can be judged by how well you look. Getting those last 5 pounds off makes the difference between looking okay and looking great. You'll lose those last 5 pounds with the No-Flab Diet, and you'll look great.

WILL I FEEL HUNGRY?

The next question a prospective dieter asks is often, "Will I feel hungry?" You'll be amazed at the amount of food you will eat on the Easy No-Flab Diet. You'll eat three medium-sized balanced meals and three snacks. And you will not be hungry.

HOW SAFE IS THE DIET?

Usually safety is one of the last concerns a person has about a diet—but the question "How Safe Is the Diet?" is the most important. Most of the health problems dieters develop come from nutrient deficiencies or energy deficiencies, that is, their blood sugar drops too low and causes problems, such as fainting. The Easy No-Flab Diet is not deficient in any nutrient and provides plenty of food energy.

Some may feel that there is too much food in the Easy No-Flab Diet. They may want to "speed things up" by omitting some foods. DO NOT OMIT any of the foods or skip any meals or snacks. That would destroy the blood-sugar stability which prevents hunger and controls fat-burning.

HOW MUCH ENERGY WILL I HAVE?

The Easy No-Flab Diet contains plenty of long-burning energy foods (100 to 105 gms of complex carbohydrates daily) spread through the day to keep blood sugar from dipping to fatigue levels. Adequate vitamins and minerals are provided to fire the energy processes and vitalize your life.

WILL I FEEL DEPRESSED?

Nearly half the dieters on conventional weight-loss programs feel depressed. The reasons include lack of diet success, B-vitamin deficiencies, lack of exercise and boredom surrounding mealtime. We now know that improper dieting can literally drive you crazy because we understand the role of protein in brain function.

Dr. Richard J. Wurtman and his associates of the Massachusetts Institute of Technology have found that several brain chemicals that control mood, learning, and hormone function are influenced by the amount of certain amino acids (the building blocks of protein) in the diet.

Serotonin, for example, is a potent regulator of brain chemistry and its deficiency causes depression. The daily

100 to 105 gm of high-quality protein in the Easy No-Flab Diet yield more than 1.5 gms of tryptophan (RDA is 0.5 gm), which influences the amount of serotonin the brain can make.

Another factor in brain function is that the mediator of nerve impulses, acetylcholine, depends on the amount of choline in the diet. The Easy No-Flab Diet is rich in choline and choline-containing lecithin. The No-Flab Diet is rich in brain fuel and all the needed brain chemicals.

WILL I FEEL STRESSED?

The No-Flab Diet produces less body stress than normal maintenance diets because it contains adequate B and C vitamins, proteins, and carbohydrates in natural whole foods.

Dr. Benjamin H. Ershoff of Loma Linda University's School of Medicine has published nearly 200 papers describing how natural foods protect the body against stress. Refined-food diets and low-carbohydrate diets, on the other hand, produce considerable mental stress and depression. The level of stress produced by a diet can be determined easily by measuring the amount of chemicals called catecholamines in the urine. The Easy No-Flab Diet gets outstanding marks. What this means is that you will remain cheerful during the diet, rather than turn mean as even the nicest people often do on other diets. The idea is to get lean, not mean.

WILL I BE CONSTIPATED?

Dieters often experience constipation because their reduced amount of food contains less food bulk, water, and B-complex vitamins than they need. The Easy No-Flab Diet provides adequate bulk, water, and B-complex vitamins, plus an exercise program to prevent sluggish bowels. If you have experienced irregularity before dieting, you will be greatly pleased to discover that No-Flab foods correct that problem.

WILL I BE ABLE TO SLEEP?

Low-carbohydrate diets often cause sleeplessness due to nutrient deficiencies. The Easy No-Flab Diet is rich in these nutrients plus the amino acid tryptophan, which helps promote restful sleep. The estimated 30 million insomniacs would all benefit from the Easy No-Flab Diet and exercise program. The restful sleep also helps keep you energized and full of pep.

WILL MY HAIR FALL OUT?

Drs. Detlef K. Goette and Richard B. Odon of the Letterman Army Medical Center in San Francisco reported that women losing more than 25 pounds in three weeks on crash diets lost hair by the handfuls. The severe calorie restriction of their crash diets deprived their hair roots of energy (*Journal of the American Medical Association*, July 1976). I suspect a vitamin B-5 (pantothenic acid) deficiency also played a role in the hair loss.

Fortunately, the Easy No-Flab Diet provides optimal energy and the nutrients needed to burn this energy. Plus, as a bonus to your hair, the diet is rich in the amino acid cystine, which is the principal component of hair protein.

The No-Flab Diet is also rich in the B-complex vitamin biotin, which helps prevent male pattern baldness because it destroys the debris from the male hormone testosterone that clogs receptors in the scalp.

The Easy No-Flab Diet provides adequate amounts of linoleic acid, an essential fat, to give the hair a beautiful sheen and gloss.

WILL MY SKIN WRINKLE OR SAG?

Very-low-calorie diets burn the lean tissue that supports facial features and your overall figure. When fat beneath the skin and lean tissue are both burned, the result is "diet sag" and deep wrinkles. Low-carbohydrate diets that produce "acid" blood (ketosis) can cause skin eruptions and cloudy, blemished skin. Vitamin deficiencies can cause dry skin and dull the sparkle in your eyes. Skin is fed from the inside, not from the outside with creams.

Fat is required to transport the fat-soluble skin vitamins A and E. Linoleic acid, the essential fat, is required for healthy skin.

Quality proteins and vitamin C are required to build the skin protein collagen. The B-vitamin niacin also helps prevent dry and patchy skin. Without adequate amounts of these nutrients, the skin sags and fingernails become brittle. The Easy No-Flab Diet is rich in nucleic acids, which some doctors believe have an anti-wrinkling effect.

The Easy No-Flab Diet will make your skin radiant and younger-looking.

DIET DESIGN

5 THE EASY NO-FLAB DIET SATISFIES BOTH the dieter and nutritionist because it allows steady fat-loss without health or emotional compromises. Before we examine how the diet preferentially sheds fat instead of the lean tissue sacrificed in numerous other diets, let's look at the basic nutrition of maintenance and reducing diets.

The body needs about fifty nutrients every day. Listed according to quantity needed, they are water, macronutrients (proteins, fats, and carbohydrates) and micronutrients (vitamins and minerals). Whether or not you're dieting, you need these nutrients. Yet most nutritionists and physicians underemphasize the need for water, vitamins, and minerals while arguing over the proper proportions of carbohydrates, fats, and proteins.

PROTEINS—THE REGULATORS OF LIFE CHEMISTRY

Our bodies are comprised mostly of water, but proteins are the nutrients next in abundance. Muscles, organs, skin, hair, teeth, and bone are made of protein, as are the life-chemistry regulators, the hormones and enzymes. Proteins can be converted by the body into fat or carbohydrates. Without protein in our diet, we would soon die.

The Recommended Daily Allowance (RDA) for protein is 56 gms (about 2 oz) for men and 46 gm for women (higher for pregnant or lactating women). However, Dr. Nevin S. Scrimshaw, Head of the Department of Nutrition and Food Science at the Massachusetts Institute of Technology, believes that the RDAs for protein are too low (*Journal of the American Medical Association*, November 21, 1977).

The average American adult eats about 100 gm (about three-and-one-half ozs) of protein a day, which is also the amount in the Easy No-Flab Diet.

FAT—THAT'S NOT WHAT MAKES YOU FAT

Fat in the diet is not the evil culprit it's made out to be. You don't have to eat fat to get fat. Too much of anything makes you fat.

On an equal weight basis, fat has more than twice the calories of protein or carbohydrates, so you do have to be careful about how much fat you eat. But fat is essential. It is required to transport the fat-soluble vitamins A, D, E, and K through the intestinal wall.

At least one polyunsaturated fatty acid (linoleic acid) is essential to life and is required in the daily diet at a level of 2 to 4 percent of total calories. Linoleic acid is widely distributed in most fats in most foods including vegetables, nuts, and whole milk.

Just as important, fat adds satiety and taste to foods, and seems to be the strongest factor in relieving hunger. Dr. E. Cheraskin and his colleagues at the University of Alabama have determined that people on moderate-fat diets have fewer medical problems than people on low-fat diets. Also, fat is required for glossy hair and smooth skin.

CARBOHYDRATES—OUR ENERGY SOURCE

Carbohydrates (often called carbos) provide quick energy. Sugars are simple-structured molecules of carbohydrates that enter the bloodstream rapidly in a form readily burned for energy. Sudden floods of sugars in the bloodstream can overwhelm the blood-sugar control mechanism. Starches and other complex carbohydrates, such as bread and potatoes, digest more slowly, eventually are converted to a sugar *but* trickle into the bloodstream over a long period of time in a more orderly process.

When we eat more carbohydrates than we require for our immediate energy needs, the excess is converted to fat and stored as fat. Since carbohydrates serve essentially little other purpose than the production of energy that can be obtained from fat or protein, they are considered the elastic or variable portion of the diet that can be adjusted to keep energy intake balanced with energy expenditures. Under ideal circumstances, proteins are conserved from energy production for their more important functions until the carbohydrates are expended.

Although the Food and Nutrition Board of the National Research Council has not established an RDA for carbohydrates, most people feel best when they get at least 100 gm (400 calories' worth) of carbohydrates daily. Most low-carbohydrate diets recommend holding the amount of carbohydrates to fewer than 60 gm daily. But that's really not enough to avoid a host of potential problems such as weakness, fatigue, irritability, and many other problems including insomnia.

FLAB CONCEPT BEATS THE CALORIE CONCEPT

In evaluating foods to determine their suitability in diets, more information is required than just how many calories are in the food. We need to know even more than the nutrient density of the food—that is, the amount of vitamins and minerals per calorie in the food. We need to know which foods set up the body chemistry necessary to stimulate fat-burning.

The proteins and carbohydrates must be considered in terms of their subclassifications, because each subclass plays a different role in fat-burning and fat-storage, as well as in hunger control.

As an example, instead of just looking at the protein content of the diet, we should first determine how much of the protein is digestible. Teeth, bone, hair, and fingernails are all protein, but not digestible. Some proteins in foods are more digestible than others.

Next we need to know how much of the digestible protein is of animal origin, because animal and vegetable proteins have slightly different body-repair and body-energy efficiencies, and because they have differing amino acid balances.

Finally for proteins, the quality must be determined in terms of their Protein Efficiency Ration (PER) or Net Protein Utilization (NPU), both of which are determined experimentally, as explained in Chapter 2. Carbohydrates are given a similar examination as to the number of FLAB Units they contain.

THE EASY NO-FLAB DIET IS A LOW INSULIN RELEASE DIET

The FLAB Index and FLAB Units obtained by this process tell us at a glance all the information needed to judge the overall chemistry of a food in terms of its suitability for shedding body fat.

The aim of the FLAB concept is to eliminate from the diet the poor-quality foods that upset the ideal blood sugar and insulin relationship, which promotes fat-burning without hunger.

The Easy No-Flab Diet is constructed to be a delicious, filling, varied diet, with approximately 1,200 well-chosen calories daily, having a minimum of 60 gm of protein, and with few sugars.

The proportions of macro-nutrients in the No-Flab Diet are approximately 35 percent protein, 35 percent carbohydrate, and 30 percent fat. There is plenty of room for variation as long as good foods are used. If you eat good foods at the right times to keep your blood sugar high enough, you'll never feel hungry.

The Easy No-Flab Diet will help you take command of your body chemistry to achieve quick and lasting fat-loss. During the diet your body chemistry will adjust from a fat person's body chemistry, which stores fat, to a thin person's body chemistry, which will make you slim and keep you naturally slender.

WHY CALORIES DON'T COUNT

IT'S NOT SIMPLY HOW MUCH YOU EAT that causes you to gain fat—it's what you eat! Few people realize that the composition of the food we eat plays the major role in establishing the body conditions that will or will not burn stored fat, because they have been misled by the calorie theory into thinking that only calorie content or the quantity of food they eat is important. Obviously, we need to know what foods will permit fat-burning if we are to design a diet that will help us get rid of flab.

One of the shortcomings of the calorie-counting theory in dieting is that it neglects the fact that body chemistry requires more energy to mobilize fat for burning than it does to store fat. It's easier to put on fat than to take it off.

Calorie information alone is adequate to tell us whether or not our food intake is below our energy needs, putting us in a situation in which we will have to burn body tissue to make up the energy deficit. But, calorie information alone will not tell us which tissues will be burned for the needed energy. The body simply does not burn fat exclusively to make up this deficit. In fact, under certain conditions it will burn relatively little fat.

47

WHY THE FOOD CALORIE IS A MISLEADING MEASURE

The calorie is a unit of heat energy, and food calories can be measured directly from the heat produced by the burning food in a calorimeter. Why do we measure food energy by burning? Because we haven't invented a machine that digests food and measures the energy available for the normal chemical reactions of the body.

Our bodies run at 98.6°F., not at the 4000°F. of a hydrocarbon-oxygen flame. Our fuel doesn't burn in a flame to release its energy of combustion; our fuel releases small amounts of energy at each of the multitude of enzymatically controlled steps, as larger compounds are processed into smaller compounds.

Our energy isn't released suddenly; food is first chewed, digested into smaller chemical units, absorbed, and then transported to cells that may *build* cell components or enzymes out of the food units, or break them down into smaller units to yield energy and waste products. We even have to produce the energy to carry out these processes. The calorimeter gets extra energy from the electrical ignition. The calorimeter burns the nitrogen in proteins, whereas we discard nitrogen in urea, creatine, or other similar compounds.

THE SPECIFIC DYNAMIC ACTION EFFECT CHALLENGES THE CALORIE THEORY

A principle developed by Dr. J. Rubner in the late nineteenth century has been used by several physicians to challenge the calorie theory. Dr. Rubner determined the basal metabolism of the man he was testing, then fed him, on separate occasions, three different diets. One of the diets was completely protein, a second was all carbohydrate, and the third was totally fat. Under fasting conditions, the man being tested burned 2,040 calories a day. When fed 2,450 calories of sugar, the man's metabolism increased slightly to 2,087 calories. This left 363 calories of sugar in his body, presumably stored as a tenth of a pound of fat. Next, the man was fed 2,450 calories of meat, and his metabolism jumped to 2,566 calories a day, thereby creating a deficit of 116 calories.

Thus on a sugar diet, the man gained weight; while on a meat diet of the same calorie content, he lost weight. Try to explain this reality with the calorie theory!

Later, another scientist found that feeding a person 100 calories' worth of protein produced more calories of body heat than 100 calories' of carbohydrates. Much has been made of this fact, called Specific Dynamic Action (SDA), to show fault with the calorie theory.

Protein, compared with carbohydrate, requires many more steps to metabolize; thus proteins require much more energy to be burned for fuel. Some of the protein that is eaten is used to repair and build tissues, while the protein that is burned for energy, uses up some energy in the process.

KETONE EXCRETION

Very-low-carbohydrate diets (which many high-protein diets are) cause a metabolic change that excretes considerable amounts of incompletely burned fats called ketones.

Many low-carbohydrate diet proponents believe this excretion of ketones removes a significant amount of stored fat from the body over and above the calories released as energy. The extra calories removed are contained in the ketones that are excreted. However, recent measurements have shown that the process of ketone excretion can account for only 100 or so calories a day, and is not a significant factor. (Dr. George Cahill, *Journal of the American Medical Association,* 1973.)

This small amount of extra excreted calories has more risk than benefit because of the side effects of ketosis, such as fatigue, weakness, dizziness, irritability, insomnia, and in rare cases, coma.

Although ketone excretion may not be so significant a factor as many believe, it still shows that the calorie theory is inefficient for describing weight-loss.

CALORIE-CANCELING FOODS

Some foods appear to use up more energy than they give the body, because the energy required to chew and digest them is greater than the energy that can be extracted from them. Foods of this type are fibrous or leafy vegetables such as celery, carrots, bean sprouts, lettuce, cabbage, and some poorly digested foods such as corn and peanuts.

Several popular diets have been designed around such "calorie-canceling" foods. Although such foods may indeed add bulk without appreciable net energy being added to the body, a diet based on such foods leaves the dieter very hungry because these foods contribute little to maintain the proper blood-sugar level. Hunger is not quenched by merely having a full stomach. Hunger is determined in the brain, not in the stomach. Stomach fullness is only part of the information the appetite control center in your brain uses to judge whether or not it should send out the "hunger" signal.

Calorie-canceling foods are usually hard and tough, so they are poorly digested. If your teeth or digestive system are less than perfect, foods such as peanuts, corn, and raw carrots may pass through you unchanged. These foods are excellent for snacks to satisfy the urge to chew, so they have great value in a diet program when used in moderation. But a diet built around such foods would be seriously deficient in essential nutrients. In any event, they illustrate a shortcoming in the calorie-counting approach.

SERIOUS FLAWS IN THE CALORIE-COUNTING CONCEPT

The calorie-counting concept is flawed because it doesn't take into account several important factors: Specific Dynamic Action, the digestibility of foods, and the net energy produced. But these are only minor flaws.

The major flaw is that the calorie concept is too general and doesn't apply to the conditions required for the mobilization of stored body fat. The calorie concept implies that when insufficient calories are eaten, the body will mobilize the calories stored as fat first, before mobilizing those stored as protein in essential tissues. This is just not the case.

Several investigators have found that during total fasting, 59 to 66 percent of the weight-loss is lean tissue.* The little fat that is lost comes mostly from the protective cushion of fat around the organs, rather than from the disfiguring fat beneath the skin.

---

*The results of Dr. F. L. Benoit and his colleagues are typical. They found that low-carbohydrate diets produced twice the fat-loss of starvation diets. In one experiment, a 10-day fast produced an average weight-loss of 20 pounds. But, only 7 of those 20 pounds were pounds of fat!

By contrast, a low-carbohydrate diet (4 percent carbohydrate) produced an average weight-loss of 13 pounds. At first glance, this diet wouldn't seem so good as the fast, because more weight was lost on the fast. The important thing, however, is that the low-carbohydrate diet produced an average of 12.6 pounds of fat-loss in the 10 days compared with the 7 pounds of fat-loss produced by the fast.

Looking at the data in another way, only 0.4 pounds of vital lean tissue was lost on the low-carbohydrate diet compared with the 13 pounds of necessary lean tissue lost on the fast. The calorie theory would predict the same fat-loss ratios for both diets, but instead we find the performance of the low-carbohydrate diet 60 times better than the fast in terms of fat-tissue to lean-tissue loss. (Annuals of Internal Medicine, 1965; Archives of Internal Medicine, 1968.)

IT'S NOT HOW MANY CALORIES YOU EAT THAT CAUSES YOU TO GAIN FAT

Dr. Rachel Schemmel of Michigan State University recognized that it's not how many calories you eat that determines fat-production or fat-burning, so much as it is how many of the different kinds of calories you eat. Dr. Schemmel found that *sugar caused greater weight gain* than an equal number of calories of whole grain cereals. Those laboratory animals eating simple-carbohydrate meals (sugar) became much fatter than those getting the complex-carbohydrate meals (starch). (*Food Product Development*, July/August 1975.)

In 1971, the uselessness of the calorie theory in fat-loss was conclusively proven by Drs. C. M. Young, S. S. Scanlan, and H. Im. They showed that college students on diets equal in number of calories and grams of protein lost fat and weight better with the least amount of carbohydrate in the diet. The more carbohydrate in the diet, the less fat they lost, even though they ate no more calories. Just as there can be too few carbohydrates, there can be too many carbohydrates in a reducing diet if you are more interested in losing fat than just pounds. Food composition is of primary importance in determining the amount of fat-loss.

In Chapter 9, you will see that the timing and distribution of meals throughout the day is just as important as the number of calories and the type of calories you eat. A given number of calories lumped into one meal may make you flabby, whereas the same number of calories spread into three meals of equal size during your periods of greatest activity may keep you slender.

It's not only how many calories you eat that causes you to gain fat. If you feel that you don't really eat that much food, then the problem is what you eat and when you eat it.

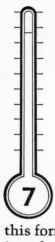

STOPPING HUNGER

7 STRANGE AS IT SOUNDS, YOU CAN STOP hunger sensations by pressing on a certain region of your ear. Yes, I said ear. We'll discuss this form of "acupressure" at the end of this chapter, but in order to lose fat you'll need to be able to do more than just relieve the symptoms of hunger: you'll need to be able to remove the cause of hunger.

No diet can be successful if it leaves dieters hungry. Low-calorie diets usually leave dieters so hungry they have to break their diets. Even "balanced" low-calorie diets will keep hunger pangs constantly gnawing at dieters' insides for several weeks while their hunger-control centers (appestat) slowly readjust to their new eating habits. Unfortunately, few people, probably less than 10 percent of us, have the willpower to resist hunger that long.

Low-carbohydrate diets, by contrast, quench the hunger pangs in a day or two, and the resulting research into why this happens has been the major contribution of the low-carbohydrate diet to the science of dieting.

Today, a newer and even better understanding of the hunger-control center and its triggers shows that we can control hunger just as quickly while dieting without experiencing the hazards of the low-carbohydrate diet.

The Easy No-Flab Diet is based on this newer understanding of the hunger-control center. It will help you lose fat without hunger—even during the first days of the diet. During the first day or two, 15 to 20 percent, mostly the more overweight-dieters, will experience slight hunger. These people will find that the ear acupressure technique will control that hunger. Most people will find the Easy No-Flab Diet so satisfying, they won't experience hunger at any point during the diet.

HUNGER AND FAT-STORAGE

When blood sugar drops below a critical level, hunger is triggered. Hunger is a natural mechanism to encourage you to eat and bring your blood-sugar level back up to preferred levels.

Whenever the blood-sugar level exceeds a certain point, as after a large meal or sugary snack, insulin is released to lower the level by speeding the conversion of blood sugar to fat. When fat is being formed, fat cannot be removed from fat cells and burned. If you wish to avoid hunger and burn fat, you should eat foods that are not very insulin-stimulating.

Each food has a different influence on the rate of insulin release. The insulin-release effects of food have been measured, and they very closely approximate the values I have determined mathematically and termed FLAB Units.

The Easy No-Flab Diet maintains the optimal blood-sugar level without stimulating the release of excessive insulin, which would cause your body to store fat. Adequate blood-sugar levels are provided by appropriate amounts of complex carbohydrates, and insulin is kept in check by the careful selection of foods that are non- or low-insulin-stimulating. Your body is maintained in a fat-burning situation. Thus you have a "thin person's" body chemistry.

Just a few poor-quality "foods" such as candy, cookies, or cakes (which have low FLAB Indexes) will disrupt the whole diet. As little as 5 percent of these poor-quality foods in the diet can switch your body chemistry back to fat-storing, rather than fat-burning, giving you a "fat person's" body chemistry.

This doesn't mean you can't occasionally eat cookies once you've reached your ideal weight. You can, but one excessive flood of insulin and the blood sugar level gyrates up and down for days in those people who tend to gain weight easily, causing hunger pangs and fat deposits. So for dieters, candy and cookies are out.

THE TROUBLESOME CARBOHYDRATES

Our problems of overweight may have started with the beginning of agriculture some 15,000 years ago. With that new development, people grew grain supplies, which could be stored. Complex carbohydrates such as corn and wheat became available in quantities that our ancestors were not equipped to handle—nor are we today.

Dr. George Christakis of Miami University theorizes that our insulin-secretion mechanism was unprepared for this carbohydrate load, and obestiy may have been the result (*Canadian Journal of Medicine*, 1967).

If the relatively slow development of agriculture was a sudden shock to our body chemistry, imagine the havoc that the sudden shift from natural foods to sweetened, processed foods has caused in our bodies. In just a few decades, which is an insignificant fraction of human history, we have changed from a diet of absolutely no processed foods and little refined sugar to a diet that contains more than 50 percent processed foods and over 100 pounds of the various refined sugars per year.

Probably because our body chemistry has been disrupted so that we crave even more sweets and junk foods, we have decided to refine from our foods the nutrients that could help stabilize our gyrating blood-sugar levels. And we have developed the habit of avoiding the high-quality foods that would get us back on the right track.

With our body chemistry so messed up, we lack energy and sit around more, so that we burn fewer calories and therefore need to eat less. When we start cutting back on calories to avoid gaining weight, we often decide to cut out the high-quality foods we need and eat the sweet stuff to satisfy the hidden hunger of our "sweet tooth."

At each step in this vicious cycle it becomes harder to get back to a good diet. It's easy enough to see that all we have to do is to replace the junk food with satisfying, nourishing—even delicious—wholesome food, and the cycle would be broken. The problem is we get hooked by the sweets. The wild gyrations of the blood-sugar levels lead to addiction ("carboholism").

We start digesting carbohydrates, simple and complex, the moment we bite into food. Saliva digests the starch in complex carbohydrates, such as those in bread, potatoes, and pastas, into smaller compounds. Enzyme action in the intestine splits these compounds into simple sugars. Within two hours, the digestible portions of complex carbohydrates have entered the blood.

Fortunately, the sugar produced from the digestion of complex carbohydrates does not enter the bloodstream all at once to overload the system as simple carbohydrates such as refined sugar do. One enzymatic reaction in the intestine splits table sugar into two simple components, which are absorbed into the blood immediately.

The blood-sugar level rises faster immediately after eating carbohydrates than after eating proteins or fat, and later, it falls faster. This is why we feel hungry again soon after a vegetarian or Chinese meal containing little meat.

THE VILLAIN—REFINED SUGAR

The sudden rise in blood sugar that occurs when refined sugar such as table sugar is eaten first produces an energy "high" and twenty minutes to an hour later produces a depressing "low" as excessive insulin floods the bloodstream and removes too much blood sugar. Before the insulin flow can be shut off, it "overshoots" and removes so much sugar that hunger results. Then you crave another "shot" of sugar, and all the while you are making fat.

Sugars such as fruit sugar that occur naturally in foods are distributed in a matrix of other nutrients that are slow digesting. Natural unrefined sugars such as fruit sugar (fructose) and milk sugar (lactose) can be handled by the body if they are eaten in moderation. These sugars as they occur in foods are diffused throughout the foods and are not absorbed into the bloodstream so rapidly as the refined sugar that has been mechanically mixed with packaged foods to sweeten them. Milk sugar is dispersed within the protein, which slows its release. This contrasts with the sugar that may be added to a fluid (such as milk) where the sugar remains in solution but not integrated within other food components.

Despite its fat-storing simulus, sugar is added to nearly all processed foods, and some people even add more sugar.

THE GLUCOSE TOLERANCE FACTOR HELPS REGULATE HUNGER

The Glucose Tolerance Factor (GTF), which is present in a number of foods, helps insulin regulate hunger. The Easy No-Flab Diet contains adequate GTF-rich foods, such as whole grain bread, cheese, and beef to fine-tune the insulin—blood-sugar balance, which is the trigger mechanism of the hunger-control center.

HUNGER FIGHTING FOODS

Proteins, fats, and fiber also aid in controlling hunger. The amino acid tryptophan, found in many proteins, helps regulate hunger (Dr. Richard Wurtman, *Journal of the American Medical Association*, 2262, 1977). Hamburger is a better hunger fighter than donuts because protein satisfies hunger longer than carbohydrates.

Fibrous foods also help control hunger. The Easy No-Flab Diet features plenty of corn because corn is a good food and supplies more fiber than originally thought by nutritionists, yet has fewer usable calories than once thought. Notice the good FLAB Index rating of an ear of corn (81.2).

Just as calories have been determined incorrectly all these years because they are calculated in a system completely unrelated to the way in which the body digests food and the way in which food nutrients are used in the body, the method for determining fiber is currently wrong.

Most of the tables listing the fiber content of foods, list values determined by grinding the foods and "digesting" them with laboratory acids and alkalies. The residue is labeled indigestible fiber. Newer analysis using digestive enzymes in simulated stomach acid and intestinal fluid mixtures has yielded vastly different results.

As an example, corn was formerly listed as having 2 percent indigestible fiber, whereas it has now been shown to be 12 percent indigestible fiber. The older method "digested" the hemicellulose and lignin, which your stomach and mine can do only very poorly.

Complex carbohydrates are very important to the dieter because they add bulk to prevent constipation and give a feeling of fullness and satiety. This is why I have added popcorn as an evening snack in the first 2 weeks of the Easy No-Flab Diet.

Dr. G. B. Haber examined the satiety value of seven

test meals all having the same calorie value (*Lancet* 1977). He had the test subjects rate their hunger or satiety on a numerical scale at intervals throughout a 3-hour test period after meals, on separate occasions, of apples, apple puree, and apple juice. Though each meal had the same number of calories, greater and longer-lasting satiety was reported with apple puree than with apple juice, and still greater satiety was reported with raw apples.

Most diets based on the calorie concept do not consider satiety, whereas the Easy No-Flab Diet based on the FLAB Unit concept does. Not feeling hungry is a critical factor in determining whether you can stay with a diet and lose fat. Thus, increasing the amount of fiber in the diet limits the tendency to overeat. And there's plenty of fiber in the Easy No-Flab Diet.

SUREFIRE HUNGER STOPPER

During your first 2 dieting days while your blood sugar and insulin are reaching homeostasis, you may find you are one of the 15 to 20 percent who will experience slight hunger sensations. If this happens, you can make them disappear by applying finger pressure at one of two points close to your ears.

Now this is not black magic, but a proven technique successfully used by three physicians on thousands of patients: Dr. Robert E. Williner of Miami, Florida, who has taught over a thousand patients how to instantly halt hunger; Dr. Keith Kenyon of Van Nuys, California, the author of *Pressure Points: Do It Yourself Acupuncture Without Needles* (Arco, 1977); and Dr. Albert Fields of the State of California's Board of Medical Assurance have all used the technique successfully.

One of these two methods will work for you. The first is to insert your index fingers gently into your ears with your palms turned toward your face. Place your thumbs on the tragus, the little bump of cartilage at the front of your external ear (not the large lobes at the bottom of your ear). Firmly massage the tragus between your thumbs and index fingers for at least a minute.

The second method is to place your index fingers in the small depressions immediately in front of your ears, just slightly higher than the tragus. Rub in a circular motion for at least one minute. (See Figure 7-1.)

I learned of this trick from an article by Ron Haines (*National Enquirer*, May 1978), and it worked for me. Try it the next time you're hungry.

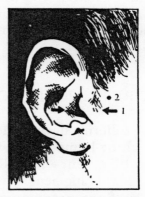

Figure 7-1 Ear Pressure Points to Control Hunger

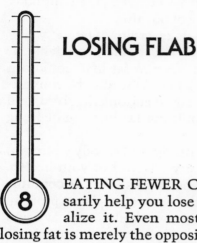

LOSING FLAB

EATING FEWER CALORIES WON'T NECES-
sarily help you lose fat. But not many people realize it. Even most nutritionists believe that
losing fat is merely the opposite of gaining fat.

Since the body can feed on its muscle as well as on its
fat, eating less can cause you to lose mostly muscle or
other lean tissue. In fact, lean-tissue loss can account for
two thirds of a dieter's weight-loss. No matter how heavy
you are, it's not essential lean tissue you should be losing.

The Easy No-Flab Diet controls conditions so your
blood sugar and insulin dictate that the weight you lose
is fat.

TAKING FAT OFF IS HARDER THAN PUTTING IT ON

It makes little difference how fast you put weight on,
but it makes a lot of difference how fast you take it off.
Your body can only burn a limited amount of fat each
day. This limit is controlled by calorie deficit, activity

61

level, and heredity factors. You can control only two of the factors. And once your calorie intake has been reduced to the limit for the effective conversion of body fat to energy, any further calorie reduction will only cause your lean tissue to be burned. You can't make your body burn more fat than it's capable of burning.

The body is unable to burn its reservoir of fat at "will," even though there are pounds and pounds available. It would be great if this could happen. A fat man could run a very long distance, if all his fat could readily be converted to energy. But there are many reactions involved, and the chemicals required for burning fat just aren't lying around waiting to be used.

Crash diets promote the burning of the body's protein, and that situation is potentially harmful to your health. But the Easy No-Flab Diet is not a crash diet. It contains adequate protein to prevent the burning of tissue protein. It is designed to pare fat from your body and leave you with a firm figure, rather than destroy your lean tissue and leave you with blobs of unshapely fat. This is what happens so often. You see people who tell you they've lost weight, but they still look fat. They're just smaller fat people.

FAT CELLS

Another major difference between putting fat on and taking it off is that fat cells can be created, but not destroyed.

Fat cells can be thought of as sacks that contain molecules of fat. As you grow fatter, these cells fill up with fat. If your body needs to store more fat, it forms more fat cells.

When you burn fat, molecules of fat are released from their storage sacks by enzymes. Although the sacks are empty, they are still there.

This, in itself, is no great disaster, merely the cause of a difference between gaining weight and losing it. The net effect is that once you become fat it will be easier to store fat again, and you will never be able to return to the exact freedom from fat you once had.

Since most of us really don't want to be actually skinny, or compete in the Mr. or Miss Universe contests, the added fat cells will be of little concern, once they are empty.

We need to leave enough fat in our fat cells to provide insulation, cushion our vital organs, and smooth our skin—but we don't need flab or fat-marbled muscles.

Breast tissue in women is primarily fatty tissue. By controlling the rate of fat-loss and the final percentage of body fat, women dieters can maintain breast fullness, without flab.

FAT-STORAGE

The production of fat is a vague concept even to many nutritionists and physicians. A greatly simplified overview is that when the blood-sugar level reaches a critical amount, additional blood sugar produced by the digestion of food will be removed from the blood by being converted to fat molecules called fatty acids. In turn, these fatty acids will be converted to triglyceride molecules, which will be deposited in the fat cells for storage.

FAT-BURNING

Fat-burning is not simply the reversal of these reactions. The body has a more compelling need to convert sugar to body fat than it normally does to convert body fat to energy. The enzymes are present to carry the reaction in the former direction, but not the latter. Reversing the direction requires different enzymes that are not present in sufficient quantities because the body of a fat person has had little use for the fat-burning chemicals. For a person who has a fat person's body chemistry, burning fat is harder than making one paycheck last till the next one.

Each step in the activation of stored body fat to the next chemical intermediate compound in the pathway to fat-burning can be influenced by many factors. The entire body chemistry must be geared to fat-burning, not just one factor, such as having a calorie deficit.

The amount of triglyceride that can be extracted from the fat cells is rate-limited because of its dependence on enzymes needed to assist in the reaction. The rate at which triglycerides can be converted to fatty acids is also controlled by enzymes not present in large quantities because there is little need for them in a body that is constantly storing fat.

The body is very efficient. It does not waste energy and nutrients making quantities of unneeded enzymes. The enzymes needed for faster fat-burning are not produced in quantity until the body has demonstrated a need for them for a sufficient period. Usually, it will take 2 to 3 days on the Easy No-Flab Diet to shift from fat-storage to fat-burning.

During this initial 2- to 3-day period you will lose weight primarily as a result of water-loss, while excess sugar stored in the liver is burned. Still you will not have burned lean tissue, and you won't during the rest of the Easy No-Flab Diet.

THE HAZARDS OF VERY-LOW-CARBOHYDRATE DIETS

Now let's look at an important difference between the Easy No-Flab Diet and very-low-carbohydrate diets. Diets very low in carbohydrates produce chemical residue forms called "ketone-bodies." The presence of a large number of ketone-bodies in the blood, which is called "ketosis," tends to make the blood more acid. This is usually not a dangerous condition, but often presents undesirable problems such as fatigue, weakness, dizziness, irritability, and insomnia. It puts a considerable strain on the kidneys, aggravates gout, and may, on rare occasion, produce coma.

Proponents of very-low-carbohydrate diets point out that the ketone-bodies help deaden the appetite and remove some fat before it has been completely burned, and thus before the fat can release all of its calories. These apparent advantages are exaggerated, however. Such excretion of ketone-bodies accounts for a loss of only 100 calories a day (Cahill, *Journal of the American Medical Association* 1973). The appetite is best controlled by developing a constant and proper level of blood sugar, and by resetting the appestat (hunger-control center)—not by putting the body in a state of ketosis.

ADVANTAGES OF THE EASY NO-FLAB DIET

The Easy No-Flab Diet doesn't produce ketone-bodies because it provides 100 to 105 gm of primarily complex carbohydrates daily. (Very-low-carbohydrate diets contain fewer than 60 gm of carbohydrates daily.) The blood-sugar level is regulated so that fatty acids follow the proper chemical pathway, rather than producing ketone-bodies.

No diet will work if you can't stay on it long enough to lose the flab *and* adjust your eating habits. The Easy No-Flab Diet is easily expanded, once you have shed all the flab you need to lose, to a perfect maintenance diet to *keep* the fat off.

HOW OFTEN SHOULD YOU EAT?

9 HOW OFTEN YOU EAT IS JUST AS IMPORtant as what you eat. Meal-timing is significant partly because it determines how well your blood-sugar level is maintained and whether or not your body develops the tendency to store excess food energy as fat.

The body responds to meal overloads and mealtime irregularity in a manner that would insure survival in a natural environment of unsure food supply. When people in prehistoric times came upon game or vegetation, they ate as much as they could because they might not feast again for some time. The unused energy from their digested food was stored as fat, which is a very compact temporary storage of food energy.

Fat enables people (and other animals) to carry around considerable amounts of calories in a convenient form. One pound of pure fat supplies the body with more than twice the number of calories of a pound of carbohydrate (3,500 vs 1,655). The storage of a pound of pure fat in fat tissue in the body can be achieved easily, because it's relatively simple to fill empty fat cells.

Unlike fat, carbohydrates, including blood sugar, can't be stored in empty sacks. Carbohydrates must be stored

66

in muscles or in the liver, and these tissues have little capacity to hold the molecules of carbohydrates. If the body could store carbohydrate in fat sacs, the blood chemistry might get very erratic.

Although 3,500 calories of fat can be stored in 1.4 pounds of fat tissue, it takes 14 pounds of lean tissue to store the same number of calories of carbohydrate. Since it's 10 times more efficient to store unneeded energy from digested food as fat, that's what the body does.

Our early ancestors depended on fat storage for survival. Today, we have a constant supply of food at our fingertips, and there is less need for body food storage. It makes more sense to store our food in refrigerators than around our waists. Storing that extra fat around our waist takes about eight hundred dollars per year extra.

EATING FEWER MEALS ISN'T THE ANSWER

Dr. Paul Fabry, a Czech nutritionist, studied the relationship between meal frequency and body-weight in 440 men. He found that there were twice as many overweight men among those who ate three or less meals a day than among those who ate five or more meals. Dr. Fabry also found the highest incidence of heart disease among the men who ate three or fewer meals per day.

ONE MEAL A DAY WON'T MAKE YOU THIN

We have known for more than a quarter of a century that one-meal-a-day eaters have more fat-producing enzymes in their bodies owing solely to this poor eating habit (V. C. Dickerson, *Yale Journal of Biology and Medicine* 1943).

We have also known for more than 20 years that the one-meal-a-day eating pattern greatly increases the efficiency of making body fat (J. Tepperman and A. Tepperman, *American Journal of Physiology* 1958).

The "stuff and starve" eating plan won't help you lose weight, even though you may eat fewer calories. It will only make you look stuffed, while you starve for most of the day. The only thing that you will lose is your temper.

SKIPPING BREAKFAST WON'T MAKE YOU THIN

Nearly as harmful as the one-meal-a-day habit is the two-meal-a-day pattern. Most people with this habit skip breakfast, have a small lunch, and then eat 70 to 80 percent of their food in the evening *when they are less active.*

Does it make sense to eat all that food when you won't have a need for its energy until the next day? Does it make sense to start off the day with no food? Not when you realize the consequences.

What is particularly disturbing, is that the body adapts to this "night eating syndrome" of the one- or two-meal-a-day eaters with changes in body chemistry that perpetuate the bad habit (Stunkard, A. J., et al., *American Journal of Medicine* 1955).

Dr. Gilbert A. LeVeille, chairman of the Department of Food Science and Human Nutrition at Michigan State University, has studied the differences in body fat between one-meal-a-day and nibbling laboratory animals for some time. He concluded in *Nutrition Today* (1975):

> People who nibble all day and forego main meals are not likely to get fat. Our experimental evidence indicates that by adhering to meal times, man has become the architect of his own obesity. Meal-eaters (three meals a day or less) stretch their larger stomachs and intestines to accommodate the extra volume and

this means a correspondingly higher *rate* of absorption of food.

Meal-eaters tend to convert carbohydrate to fat immediately. They build up a high degree of rapid efficiency in this conversion and develop a sluggishness in the reverse direction.

Dr. LeVeille also noted that "Only man and his domesticated pets are geared to regular meals and they are the only ones that have a problem with obesity."

THE TEST THAT PROVED IT

Dr. Barbara Edelstein reports in her book, *The Woman Doctor's Diet for Women* (Prentice Hall, 1977), a study in which four meal patterns were compared. One group ate a 250-calorie breakfast, a 250-calorie lunch, and a 500-calorie dinner. The group averaged about 2 pounds of weight-loss per week on the three-meal, 1,000-calorie-a-day diet.

A second group skipped breakfast, ate a 250-calorie lunch, and a 500-calorie dinner. How much more weight did the second group lose? Not a bit more. The second group, although they ate 250 fewer calories, also averaged about 2 pounds per week loss.

A third group—poor souls—was put on one 500-calorie meal a day. They ate the same dinner as the first two groups that lost an average of 2 pounds a week, but the third group skipped breakfast and lunch. How much weight did the third group lose? (The group ate 3,500 calories less than group one per week.) Well, the third group averaged the same weight-loss as the first two groups—about 2 pounds a week!

A fourth group was also put on the "stuff and starve" one-meal-a-day diet, but they were allowed a 1,000-calorie dinner. How much did group four lose? Wrong! They lost less than 1 pound a week on the average.

This really shoots the old calorie theory to smith-ereens.

Dr. Edelstein later repeated this experiment with comparable results, except in her experiment, the fourth group didn't lose any weight. It seems that the size of the dinner meal and number of meals eaten does have a major role in weight control. And there are other reasons for avoiding large meals. They produce more heart attacks and speed the aging process.

BIG BREAKFASTS AND EARLY LUNCHES ASSIST IN FAT-LOSS

A study by the U.S. Army Research and Development Command at Natick, Massachusetts, led by Drs. Ronald Gatty and Curtis Graeber, found that a big breakfast or early lunch benefited weight-loss. Dr. Gatty advised, "You must leave time to work off the calories. Evening calories turn to fat."

IMPORTANCE OF BREAKFAST

With the importance of several small meals spaced throughout the day established, let's look at typical American breakfasts.

Ten percent of Americans skip breakfast completely, while a good percentage have just coffee alone or coffee plus toast or a Danish. That's no meal. Even cereal and milk is short of a substantial meal. You should breakfast like a king.

THE EASY NO-FLAB DIET PROVIDES SEVERAL MEALS

The Easy No-Flab Diet provides a hearty breakfast plus a midmorning snack. You will be happy and alert all morning and enjoy your snack, instead of craving a "pick-up" at the "coffee break."

During the first few weeks of the diet (until your blood sugar and insulin have reached their desired homeostasis), you will eat several snacks a day—along with three 400-calorie meals—and you'll lose flab. You will never feel as though you are skimping on food, because you won't be.

WOMEN ARE DIFFERENT FROM MEN WHEN IT COMES TO WEIGHT-LOSS

10 MOST DIETS IGNORE THE DIFFERENCES between men and women in terms of energy needs and fat metabolism. Nearly everyone realizes that men, on the average, are larger than women and therefore have more cells to feed. Men need more food energy than women primarily because of size differences, but also because men are not insulated so well as women and hence they lose more heat energy to the environment.

Yes, women have more fat cells beneath the skin than men do. This is why women are generally softer to the touch. This extra fat acts like a blanket to keep heat in, but makes it harder for a woman to lose fat. Normal-weight women average about 26 percent of their body weight as fat, while normal-weight men average about 16 percent fat. Considering psychological and environmental factors as well, it's nearly twice as easy for men to lose fat.

In order for a man to stay on a diet long enough to lose weight, he must have adequate energy to meet his needs and comfort. In terms of calories, an active, middle-aged man would not be comfortable on fewer than 1,500 calories a day, whereas a woman could easily feel energetic on as few as 1,200 calories.

But, remember, losing FAT is more involved than just losing weight. All the factors (food quantity, food quality, frequency of eating, calorie deficit, and rate of weight-loss) must be considered. The two biggest differences between men and women affecting FAT-loss are in hormone activity and number of fat cells. Men maintain their weight with about 15 calories a day per pound of body weight, while women need only 12 calories a day per pound of body weight.

Surveys taken by the U.S. Public Health Service find that American women have their biggest weight problems following pregnancies and menopause. Men gain weight steadily between the ages of 25 and 40, and faster after 40.

IT'S HARDER FOR WOMEN TO LOSE FAT

Women have an extra layer of fat. Its purpose is to feed, heat, and protect the fetus during pregnancy, and the extra fat cells are there even when the woman is not pregnant. (During pregnancy, even more fat is stored in the cells.) This extra layer of fat does more than conserve heat energy (calories). Each fat cell is a bustling chemical factory ready to gather blood sugar and convert it to fat. If more fat factories are working at the same time, more fat is produced.

To make matters worse for fat-loss, the female hormones estrogen and progesterone are somewhat like insulin, in that they increase the rate at which molecules of blood sugar enter the fat cells. This effect is intensified in women taking birth control pills, which can increase the rate of conversion of blood sugar to fat by 10 to 20 percent, plus increase the amount of water retained in lean tissue.

Even women past menopause or those who have had a hysterectomy have sufficient levels of the female hormones to enhance the conversion of blood sugar to body fat.

Weight-gain after menopause is the result of less activity. Fatigue comes much quicker to women after menopause or after a hysterectomy because activity is limited, due to long-lasting extreme post-operative fatigue that is the outcome of the loss of so much internal tissue and a more sedentary life-style. This pattern can aggravate itself in a downward spiral. As the body fat increases, the body is better insulated against heat-loss; thus not so many calories need be burned to produce heat. And the extra weight tires the body quickly. Often eating food is used to compensate for the lack of other pleasures. The solution is to break the cycle early.

Post-menopausal women should expect some increase in breast and thigh size, but the fat increase can be stopped before fat accumulates around the waist. Taking off the extra fat is harder for post-menopausal women than for younger women, and harder for younger women than for men, but it can be done efficiently and painlessly without stress.

IT'S EASIER FOR WOMEN TO GAIN WEIGHT

In addition to the physiological (biochemical) factors that women have to contend with to lose fat, there are also psychological factors. Most women are responsible for buying and preparing food. The temptation is there to nibble while "tasting" the cooking, preparing school lunches, or dealing with leftover food so that it's not wasted.

The nearby convenience of the refrigerator is tempting for instant gratification, especially when problems occur or neighbors or friends drop in for a visit. The average housewife eats 18 times a day according to Dr. Lyn Howard, an Albany Medical College physician. Nibbling is fine, but not when combined with three large meals.

Another major psychological problem dieting women face is caused by the weight fluctuations (due to water-retention changes) during their monthly cycle. Just when the diet looks successful, and a woman has regained pride in herself, the scale shows a weight-gain. The dieter's pride is demolished; she abandons the diet and may over-eat to compensate for her unhappiness.

Or, aware of the fluid retention, a woman may decide her weight-gain is only temporary and continue to eat not knowing how much of the gain is water retention and how much is from overeating and will still be there when the menstrual cycle changes.

These weight increases can confuse a woman on a diet and at times depress her because they interrupt her dieting program. Finally, the woman may just give up. Her guilt may deepen because she feels she's failed, especially if her friends, who do not have so severe a water-retention problem, make steady progress in losing weight or staying trim.

Dieters should never feel that they are a failure at dieting. If you have a fat-storing body chemistry you will not be able to break it by willpower. It takes the knowledge given here to convert your body chemistry to fat-burning chemistry.

The Easy No-Flab Diet stresses fat-loss, not weight-loss, and whether male or female, the dieter will not be distracted by water-retention fluctuations or will-demolishing hunger.

THE DIFFERENCE IN RESPONSE TO EXERCISE

To really make it harder for women to lose weight, there is an important difference in their response to exercise. When a man exercises consistently, his *basal metabolism* (energy consumed while at rest) increases dramatically to burn more calories, even at rest.

When a woman exercises consistently, she receives little more weight-loss benefit than the burning of the calories needed to perform the exercise. (Of course, there are many other important benefits of exercise.) However, women do not have a great increase in fat-burning enzymes due to consistent exercise. Again men are luckier when it comes to losing fat.

Both men and women dieters need the benefits of regular exercise. Without exercise, it's difficult to lose fat from the key F-A-T areas (Fanny, Abdomen, and Thighs). Exercise helps shape these areas as well. An exercise program is explained in Chapters 25 and 26.

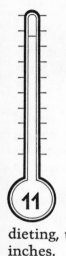

HOW MUCH
SHOULD YOU WEIGH?

11 MOST PEOPLE JUDGE WHETHER THEY should diet by how they look in the mirror or by how well their clothes fit. Yet, when they start dieting, their thoughts turn to losing pounds rather than inches.

It may be a little easier to measure pounds by stepping on the bathroom scale, but the scale tells you comparatively little. It totals lean tissue, water, and fat, when all you really need to measure is the fat. Weight-loss can be mostly water, mostly muscle, or mostly fat. The scale can't tell you which you are losing.

A survey by the A. C. Nielsen Company published in 1978 projected that nearly 42 million people had been on some kind of diet during 1977, and that well over half the women between 25 and 34 years of age had been on a diet during the previous year (*Food Product Development* June 1978).

Women continue to gain weight for longer than men, perhaps as a result of eating more to compensate for increased fatigue after menopause. Average weights of women increase rapidly until 35 to 44 years, but don't peak until 55 to 64 years.

Average weights of men increase most rapidly until 25 to 34 years of age, and eventually peak between 35 and 44 years for tall men and between 45 and 54 years for men shorter than 5 feet 8 inches, according to a 1978 survey of 10,000 persons by the National Center for Health Statistics.

A 1978 *Glamour* magazine survey to which 30,000 readers responded found that 95 percent of the women indicated they were dieting at least part of the time, with 49 percent trying to lose weight most of the time. The average woman surveyed had been on a diet 4 times.

Teen magazine polled its readers in 1977 and found that 88 percent of the 9,300 teens surveyed felt they were overweight. Only 6 percent felt their weight was just right, but many were fighting hard to hold their weight steady.

WHAT WE ACTUALLY WEIGH

According to the National Center for Health Statistics, Americans have been getting fatter. The average man surveyed from 1971 through 1974 weighed 4 pounds more than the average man in a similar survey taken a decade earlier. Women younger than 45 also averaged about 4 pounds more than their counterparts a decade earlier. Although these men and women were generally a half inch taller than their predecessors, their weight-gain was more apt to be fat than lean tissue.

The average woman surveyed was 15 to 20 pounds above her ideal weight, and the average man was 20 to 30 pounds over his ideal weight. The survey was based on measurements taken of 13,600 Americans between the ages of 18 and 74.

An earlier survey by the National Center had indicated that the average American woman puts on a pound a year from age 25 to 50.

TABLE 11-1
Actual Average Weights 1971-1974

(NOTES: These are not desirable weights. Weight includes an estimated half pound of clothing.)

Source—National Center for Health Statistics U.S. Public Health Service

Women

Height (no shoes)	Age Group 18-24	25-34	35-44	45-54	55-64	65-74
4' 9"	114	118	125	129	132	130
4' 10"	117	121	129	133	136	134
4' 11"	120	125	133	136	140	137
5' 0"	123	128	137	140	143	140
5' 1"	126	132	141	143	147	144
5' 2"	129	136	144	147	150	147
5' 3"	132	139	148	150	153	151
5' 4"	135	142	152	154	157	154
5' 5"	138	146	156	158	160	158
5' 6"	141	150	159	161	164	161
5' 7"	144	153	163	165	167	165
5' 8"	147	157	167	168	171	169

Men

Height (no shoes)	Age Group 18-24	25-34	35-44	45-54	55-64	65-74
5' 2"	130	141	143	147	143	143
5' 3"	135	145	148	152	147	147
5' 4"	140	150	153	156	153	151
5' 5"	145	156	158	160	158	156
5' 6"	150	160	163	164	163	160
5' 7"	154	165	169	169	168	164
5' 8"	159	170	174	173	173	169
5' 9"	164	174	179	177	178	173
5' 10"	168	179	184	182	183	177

Men

Height	Age Group					
(no shoes)	18–24	25–34	35–44	45–54	55–64	65–74
5' 11"	173	184	190	187	189	182
6' 0"	178	189	194	191	193	186
6' 1"	183	194	200	196	197	190
6' 2"	188	199	205	200	203	194

DESIRABLE WEIGHTS

How we see ourselves helps determine our actual weight. If we always think we look fat when we look in the mirror, we'll probably diet more and actually not be so fat as our neighbors. If when we look in the mirror, we tend to overlook a little flab, we may be heavier than our neighbors.

Basically the desired weight for a woman of medium build between the ages of 20 and 40 is 100 pounds for her first 5 feet of height and 5 pounds for each additional inch. A man can comfortably weigh 115 pounds for his first 5 feet of height and 5 pounds for each additional inch.

Individual variations are great, and some variations such as muscularity or bone structure affect weight. Many athletes, for example, are far above the ideal weight indicated by charts, yet they are in better shape than many non-athletes at the "desirable" weight, who have little muscularity.

A refinement in weight tables that helps makes them more meaningful is classification by body-frame size.

FRAME SIZE

How do you know if you are small- medium- or large-framed? Most of us think we know, but are never sure. Yet differences in the weight tables are appreciable between adjacent frame sizes.

Suppose you believe you have a medium frame, and you're struggling to get a few more pounds of fat off, when in reality you are heavy-framed and already at your ideal weight? Suppose you stopped dieting when you reached the ideal weight listed for a medium frame, and you're really small-framed? Knowing your frame size is important if you are going to rely on weight tables.

We have inherited our basic body shape. There are three major classifications: mesomorphs, endomorphs, and ectomorphs, although Dr. William Sheldon of the University of Oregon has identified eighty variations of the three basic shapes.

Mesomorphs have bodies proportioned more toward shoulder-width than stomach-width. Endomorphs have body proportions relatively broader toward stomach and hips than in the shoulders, and tend to have excess fat. Ectomorphs are relatively equally proportioned between shoulders and hips, and are slender with little excess fat (see Figure 11-2).

Often, people in the small-framed category are ectomorphs, medium-framed people are mesomorphs, and large-framed people are endomorphs.

When you compare the percentage of weight-gain by age 38 to their weight at 18 years, you find that ectomorphs average gains between 0 and 9 percent; mesomorphs between 10 and 19 percent; and endomorphs between 20 and 29 percent (see Figure 11-3).

As indicated by the percent of weight gained by age 38 compared with weight at 18 years, endomorphs put on weight more easily than ectomorphs. Adapted from Dr. Garret Peterson in *Atlas for Somatotyping Children.*

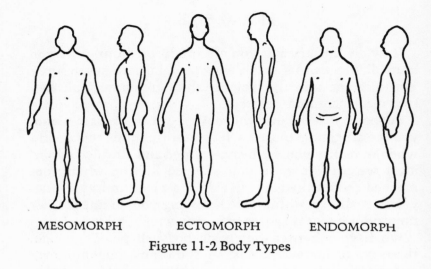

MESOMORPH   ECTOMORPH   ENDOMORPH

Figure 11-2 Body Types

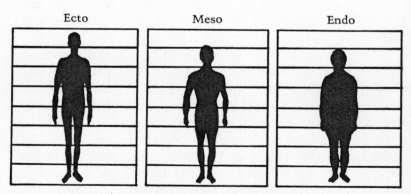

Ecto   Meso   Endo

Figure 11-3 Body Build Affects Weight Gain

DETERMINING YOUR FRAME SIZE

To help in judging which frame size you have for the purpose of using weight tables, you may check your wrist size. Encircle your wrist at its smallest circumference between the thumb and the middle finger of your opposite hand. If your finger and thumb meet or almost meet, you are probably medium-framed. If they fall short by nearly an inch or more, you are probably (but not necessarily) large-framed. If your finger and thumb overlap by more than a half inch, you are probably small-framed.

It's still a matter of subjective comparison. Consider the following: If your foot is wide, you may be large-framed; if your foot is narrow, you may be small-framed. Men, how about your hat size? Often a hat size larger than 7½ indicates a large frame, whereas a hat size smaller than 7 indicates a small frame. Women, how about your glove size? A large hand indicates a large frame. A 6½ glove size indicates a small frame.

If most of these indicators suggest primarily one frame size, the odds are that's your proper classification.

But, if you reach the desired weight indicated by the tables, and you look heavy or skinny in the mirror, go by the mirror, not the tables

FINDING YOUR DESIRABLE WEIGHT

To find your desirable weight, take measurements in your stocking feet, while wearing less than one-half pound of clothing.

Use the tables as a rough guide, but, remember, no two people are exactly alike. The amount of fat and the proportions in which fat is deposited are the result of strong genetic influence. Don't try to reach an impossible "average" desirable figure that doesn't fit your genetic background. Instead, recognize the difference, and try to improve your inherited figure to become the best it can be.

TABLE 11-4
Desirable Weights

Women

Height (no shoes)	Small	Frame Size Medium	Large
4'8"	92– 98	96–107	104–119
4'9"	94–101	98–110	106–122
4'10"	96–104	101–113	109–125
4'11"	99–107	104–116	112–128
5'0"	102–110	107–119	115–131
5'1"	105–113	110–122	118–134
5'2"	108–116	113–126	121–138
5'3"	111–119	116–130	125–142
5'4"	114–123	120–135	129–146
5'5"	118–127	124–139	133–150
5'6"	122–131	128–143	137–154
5'7"	126–135	132–147	141–158
5'8"	130–140	136–151	145–163
5'9"	134–144	140–155	149–168
5'10"	138–148	144–159	153–173

Men

Height (no shoes)	Small	Frame Size Medium	Large
5'1"	112–120	118–129	126–141
5'2"	115–123	121–133	129–144
5'3"	118–126	124–136	132–148
5'4"	121–129	127–139	135–152
5'5"	124–133	130–143	138–156
5'6"	128–137	134–147	142–161
5'7"	132–141	138–152	147–166
5'8"	136–145	142–156	151–170
5'9"	140–150	146–160	155–174
5'10"	144–154	150–165	159–179

Men

Height (no shoes)	Small	Frame Size Medium	Large
5'11"	148–158	154–170	164–184
6'0"	152–162	158–175	168–189
6'1"	156–167	162–180	173–194
6'2"	160–171	167–185	178–199
6'3"	164–175	172–190	182–204

Weights are with less than one-half pound of clothing. Adapted from tables prepared by Boehringer Ingelheim, Ltd., Elmsford, N.Y. 10523.

WEIGHT IS NOT THE BEST INDICATOR OF BODY FAT

12 WEIGHT TABLES CANNOT TAKE IN-dividual muscularity into account and give only poor consideration to body type. However, the biggest criticism of weight tables and measurements is that they confuse and discourage a dieter. The daily fluctuations in weight, due to water retention and undigested dietary bulk, often cause a dieter to abandon a diet even while fat is actually melting away.

Another problem for dieters is that the initial loss of intestinal bulk, or water-loss from exercising, may be misinterpreted as fat-loss. At that point, the overconfident dieter treats the diet program too casually, and fat-loss comes to a stop.

EVEN ATHLETES DON'T UNDERSTAND WEIGHT-LOSS AFTER EXERCISE

Athletes are often confused by their weight-loss after a workout. They feel that they have burned off fat. But the amount of body fat burned during any one exercise session is small, because each ounce of fat is so power-packed. (An ounce of fat provides about 220 calories, enough to play tennis for 20 minutes.)

Ounce for ounce, carbohydrate provides less energy than fat, so in order to play tennis for 20 minutes, you would have to burn 2½ oz of glycogen, the immediate source of energy stored as carbohydrate.

What many professional athletes don't realize is that burning 2½ oz of glycogen will release approximately 5 to 10 oz of water, making a total of 12½ oz of weight-loss.

After playing tennis for an hour, a pro or an amateur can experience a weight-loss greater than 2 pounds, not even counting water lost as perspiration. But that's only temporary. As the glycogen is replaced, water is also returned to the muscle tissue.

The net result a few hours after exercise is not the 2-pound weight-loss, but a 3-oz fat-loss.

Oh, it's a morale booster for dieters to exercise hard for a few days and deplete their glycogen stores. Their weight drops fast and they get psyched up. However, as soon as they miss exercising for a day and their glycogen levels return to normal, they may feel devastated by their increase in weight unless they understand what is happening.

DON'T MISTAKE WATER RETENTION FOR WEIGHT-GAIN

Water retention not only varies with glycogen level, but also with hormone levels and genetic differences. A 120-pound woman averages about 70 pounds of water and 50 pounds of solids. A day after she weighs-in at 120, the solids may weigh exactly the same but her water content may temporarily have increased by 5 pounds so that, although the scales register 125 pounds, she actually isn't any fatter.

The water content of individuals varies from 45.6 to

70.2 percent. You can readily see how the diuretic action of low-carbohydrate diets can cause a great weight-loss (water-loss) without appreciable fat loss. Women, because of their greater fat content, average about 10 percent lower in water content than men. A person weighing 120 pounds may contain as much as 65 pounds of solids or as little as 36 pounds.

DON'T MISTAKE FIRM MUSCLE WEIGHT FOR UNDESIRABLE WEIGHT

A State Police Officers' Association once complained to me that their department was imposing unfair physical-fitness standards on the officers based on weight tables. The problem was that many officers were weight-lifters or body-builders and were very muscular. Although they seemed too heavy according to weight charts, these officers were in better physical condition than most of the lighter weight officers and administrators who were less muscular. It's quite possible for a sedentary person of the "desired" weight to be carrying more flab than a well-conditioned athlete who seems appreciably "overweight" according to the tables.

Most athletic trainers are aware of this. As an example, every year at the beginning of summer camp, the Washington Redskins are given thorough physical and conditioning examinations, including percent-body-fat calculations based on skin-thickness measurements. Some teams even use underwater weighings to measure total body fat. (Since fat floats, the lighter you weigh underwater, the fatter you are.)

Muscle tissue is useful, attractive, and does not impose a burden on the heart. Excess fat is useless, unattractive, and forces the heart to push blood through miles of extra vessels needlessly. Table 12-1 compares the composition of muscle and fat tissues. Notice that the value for a

TABLE 12-1
Comparison of Muscle and Fat Tissue

	Water	Fat	Protein	Cals/lb
Muscle	70%	7%	22%	563
Fat	22%	72%	6%	2,505

pound of actual tissue differs from the value for a pound of pure fat or pure protein.

Keep in mind that if your body needs 2,500 more calories than is provided by your food, it can burn 4½ pounds of muscle tissue, 1 pound of fat tissue, or a combination of the two.

The Easy No-Flab Diet aims at burning the fat tissue rather than the muscle tissue, but unless we can measure fatness, we can't be sure. The following chapter will tell you how to *be* sure.

HOW TO MEASURE BODY FAT

THE MIRROR OFFERS THE EASIEST WAY
to see if you have excess fat or not, but some
people have forgotten what a good figure looks
like. If you are the trimmest in a family of fat people, you
may look "skinny" to your family. And some people let
their minds distort their mirror image. If you've forgotten
what a good figure looks like, flip through a few issues of
the magazines that show the bare waistlines of men and
women "figure" models. Or if you want to be as slim as
fashion models, look at the fashion magazines.

If your chest and waist are the same size, you're fat,
and if your waist is larger, you are considerably over your
ideal weight.

THE RULER TEST

You can measure some body fat with a ruler. Lie on
your back and rest a ruler lengthwise on your abdomen
from your rib cage to your pelvis. If your pouch tilts the
ruler so that both ends don't touch your body, you need
to reduce and/or do situps regularly. If you can't find your

pelvis . . . well, it's a good thing you're reading this book.

THE PINCH TEST

An even more accurate indicator of body fat than the scale, mirror, or ruler is the "pinch test" to measure skin-fold thickness (or fat-fold thickness). The pinch test may not be so accurate as underwater weighing, soft X rays, or potassium-40 tests, but it meets the needs of the dieter interested in losing FLAB.

Skin-fold measurements are based on the fact that the amount of fat beneath the skin is about one half the total body fat. The distribution of deposited fat in each area of the body is determined by heredity, so skin-fold measurements should be taken in several body regions: waist, back, arm, chest, leg, and buttocks.

To perform the pinch test you gently lift a fold of skin away from the soft tissue and bone by grasping the skin between the thumb and index finger. This double fold of skin also contains the fat layer beneath the skin. The measurement will be the amount of skin separating your thumb and finger, not the distance the skin is pulled away from the body. In all pinch measurements, the pinched skin fold should run in the direction of head to toe.

Next, place the points of a draftsman's caliper compass (used to draw circles) snugly on each side of the skin fold. (Be sure to first place tape over the compass point and pinch point so that you don't prick your skin.) Make all pinch-test measurements at the point at which you feel pressure or snugness from the calipers. It is better to have someone make the measurements for you, but you can do them yourself. Measure the distance between the compass points with a ruler, preferably with a millimeter or centimeter scale. Record the measurements.

THE TEST 40 PERCENT OF ALL AMERICANS FAIL

Most physicians use just one measurement on the back of the arm in the triceps region. If that pinch is between one half and one inch, you have a "normal" amount of fat (see Table 13-1). If it's more than one inch thick, you are too fat, even if your weight is appropriate for your height. If you are trim, your tricep's skin fold will be less than three quarters of an inch for men and one inch for women. More than 40 percent of all Americans fail this test.

PINCH-TEST RESULTS

So that you may monitor the disappearance of fat, I suggest one of the following two methods for taking the pinch test. Method A involves only four "pinches" but requires a partner because of the back measurement. Method B involves seven "pinches" but can be done by yourself. Method A is the more accurate test for body fat. In both methods, repeat the measurement a second time to be sure of accuracy.

For Pinch-Test Method A, total the skin-fold measurements in these four areas: the front of the upper arm at the biceps, the rear of the upper arm at the triceps, the back just below the shoulder blade, and the side of the waist. Compare your total with the totals in Table 13-2. Remember that the athletic male has less than 12 percent body fat (marathon runners around 4 percent), and trim women have around 26 percent. The average male will have 16 percent body fat, and the average female 26 percent. Men having more than 20 percent body fat, and women having more than 30 percent, are obese.

For Pinch Test Method B, more easily accessible body regions are used, but there is no large collection of data to correlate total pinch measurements vs percent body fat.

TABLE 13-1
The Test 40 Percent of All Americans Fail

If your tricep's skin fold is greater than the figure below, you are considered obese.

AGE	SKIN FOLD			
	WOMEN		MEN	
	inches	mm	inches	mm
18	1.06	27	0.59	15
20	1.10	28	0.62	16
22	1.10	28	0.71	18
24	1.10	28	0.75	19
26	1.14	29	0.79	20
28	1.14	29	0.87	22
30–50	1.18	30	0.91	23

Adapted from C. C. Seltzer and J. Mayer, "Postgraduate Medicine" 1965.

Seven measurements are taken, and if they total 9 to 9½ inches your percentage of body fat is okay. More than that means you're carrying excess body fat.

Measure your skin folds at: the forearm, side of waist, buttocks, cheek, front thigh, rear thigh, and hip.

Keep in mind that as you lose fat, at first more may come from one area than another, but soon that pattern will shift and you will lose more fat from another area. The patterns of fat-gain and fat-loss vary according to family characteristics. Eventually, the fat will disappear from all areas. I have yet to find a person with bony ribs, thin legs and face, and flat stomach and fat hips or vice versa. So be sure to measure all the areas to monitor your fat-loss.

Vincent Antonetti, author of *The Computer Diet,*

TABLE 13-2*
Percentage Body Fat—Pinch-Test Method A

Total Pinch measurements taken at biceps, triceps, back, and waist indicate the percentage body fat. Numbers in parentheses represent rounded-off values.

WOMEN		AGE			
inches	mm	16–29	30–39	40–49	50+
0.79	20	14.1	17.0	19.8	21.4
0.99 (1)	25	16.8	19.4	22.2	24.0
1.18	30	19.5	21.8	24.5	26.6
1.38	35	21.5	23.7	26.4	28.5
1.58	40	23.4	25.5	28.2	30.3
1.77	45	25.0	26.9	29.6	31.9
1.97 (2)	50	26.5	28.2	31.0	33.4
2.17	55	27.8	29.4	32.1	34.6
2.36	60	29.1	30.6	33.2	35.7
2.56	65	30.2	31.6	34.1	36.7
2.76	70	31.2	32.5	35.0	37.7
2.96 (3)	75	32.2	33.4	35.9	38.7
3.15	80	33.1	34.3	36.7	39.6
3.35	85	34.0	35.1	37.5	40.4
3.55	90	34.8	35.8	38.3	41.2
3.74	95	35.6	36.5	39.0	41.9
3.94 (4)	100	36.4	37.2	39.7	42.6
4.33	110	37.8	38.6	41.0	43.9
4.73	120	39.0	39.6	42.0	45.1
5.12	130	40.2	40.6	43.0	46.2
5.90	150	42.3	42.6	45.0	48.2
6.90	175	–	44.8	47.0	50.4
7.88	200	–	46.5	48.8	52.4

*Adapted from J.V.G.A. Durnin and J. Womersley, *British Journal of Nutrition* 1974.

MEN		AGE			
inches	*mm*	*17–29*	*30–39*	*40–49*	*50+*
0.79	20	8.1	12.2	12.2	12.6
0.99 (1)	25	10.5	14.2	15.0	15.6
1.18	30	12.9	16.2	17.7	18.6
1.38	35	14.7	17.7	19.6	20.8
1.58	40	16.4	19.2	21.4	22.9
1.77	45	17.7	20.4	23.0	24.7
1.97 (2)	50	19.0	21.5	24.6	26.5
2.17	55	20.1	22.5	25.9	27.9
2.36	60	21.2	23.5	27.1	29.2
2.56	65	22.2	24.3	28.2	30.4
2.76	70	23.1	25.1	29.3	31.6
2.96 (3)	75	24.0	25.9	30.3	32.7
3.15	80	24.8	26.6	31.2	33.8
3.35	85	25.5	27.2	32.1	34.8
3.55	90	26.2	27.8	33.0	35.8
3.74	95	26.9	28.4	33.7	36.6
3.94 (4)	100	27.6	29.0	34.4	37.4
4.33	110	28.8	30.1	35.8	39.0
4.73	120	30.0	31.1	37.0	40.4
5.12	130	31.0	31.9	38.2	41.8
5.52	140	32.0	32.7	39.2	43.0
5.90	150	32.9	33.5	40.2	44.1
6.30	160	33.7	34.3	41.2	45.1
6.70	170	34.5	34.8	42.0	46.1

Evans & Co., New York, 1973, has developed a table to give men a quick idea of their body-fat content based on their weight and waist size (see Table 13-3).

In addition to the pinch test, you should measure and record your vital statistics: the circumference of your waist, hips, chest/breast, thigh, calf, and arm.

TABLE 13-3*
Percent Body Fat for Men

Weight						
			Waist Size (inches)			
	34	36	38	40	42	44
140	22.3	28.2	34.1	–	–	–
150	20.3	25.8	31.3	–	–	–
160	18.5	23.7	28.9	34.0	–	–
170	16.9	21.8	26.7	31.5	–	–
180	15.5	20.1	24.7	29.3	33.9	–
190	14.3	18.6	23.0	27.4	31.7	–
200	13.1	17.3	21.4	25.6	29.7	33.9
220	11.2	15.0	18.7	22.5	26.3	30.1
240	9.6	13.0	16.5	19.9	23.4	26.9
260	8.2	11.4	14.6	17.8	21.0	24.2

*Adapted from *The Computer Diet*, Evans & Co., New York, 1973, by Vincent Antonetti.

To sum it up, if you can grab much flab, it should come off. And it will if you follow the easy program of the easy No-Flab Diet and Exercise Plan.

HOW FAST WILL YOU LOSE FAT?

(14) YOU WILL LOSE FAT AT A RAPID RATE. It's human nature to want to shed those pounds as fast as you can. But if you lose weight faster than your body can metabolize fat, you will also lose vital lean tissue. Women will lose figure-supporting muscles and breast tissue. Men will lose strength. If you must lose weight at breakneck speed for some legitimate reason, the Diet Shakes described in Chapter 23 can be used safely—but that quick loss will only be temporary unless you finish it off with the Easy No-Flab Diet.

The Easy No-Flab Diet is designed to melt away fat as rapidly as your body can mobilize it, while assuaging your hunger and building your energy. While the fat disappears, you learn new food habits that will prevent you from putting fat right back on.

HOW FAST YOU CAN EXPECT TO LOSE FAT

If you are more than 20-pounds overweight, you can expect to lose more than 13 pounds of fat (not counting water loss) each month on the standard No-Flab Diet.

That's more than 3 pounds of FLAB each week. A person weighing 250 who is more than 30-pounds overweight can lose 30 pounds per month.

For those with less than 20 pounds to lose, the rate will be proportionately slower. Table 14-1 shows the rate of fat-loss on the Easy No-Flab Diet.

The average woman (5 feet 3½ inches tall and weighing 143 pounds) is exactly 20-pounds overweight. On the Easy No-Flab Diet she would lose 10.5 pounds the first month, 8.5 pounds the second month and be at her desired weight in 10 weeks. She will lose 20 pounds of fat tissue at the ideal rate of 2 pounds a week.

The average man (5 feet 9 inches tall and weighing 172 pounds) is exactly 20-pounds overweight. On the Easy No-Flab Diet he will lose 13.5 pounds the first month, and be at his ideal weight in 3 more weeks. His loss of 20 pounds of fat tissue will occur in 7 weeks. As explained earlier, height and hormonal differences make it easier for men to lose fat, and 3 pounds a week for a 5-foot, 9-inch man, 20-pounds overweight is just right.

The amount of fat you lose will depend on your faithfulness to the diet, your individual biochemistry, and your present weight. If you are fatter than average, you will lose weight faster. The closer you are to your ideal weight, the longer it will take. Let's follow an example through the charts to predict the average fat-loss of a woman 32-pounds overweight. Let's assume she weighs 147 pounds—her desired weight is 115 pounds.

This woman is more than 20-pounds overweight, so she should use Table 14-1, Section A, until she weighs less than 135 pounds. When she is less than 20-pounds overweight, she should use Section B.

To estimate her weight-loss for her first month on the Easy No-Flab Diet, she should follow the weight line closest to her actual current weight (147 pounds) for 4 weeks. If at the end of 4 weeks, the woman crosses the

TABLE 14-1
Rate of Fat-Loss

Standard No-Flab Diet, Weekly Fat-Loss Averages for Men and Women

A: More than 20-Pounds Overweight

Maximum Fat-Tissue Loss (72% Fat, 22% Water, 6% Protein)

Present Weight	Week 1	Week 2	Week 3	Week 4	Total Month (4.3 weeks)
250	7.1	6.8	6.6	6.3	28.9
240	6.7	6.4	6.2	5.9	27.2
230	6.3	6.0	5.8	5.5	25.4
220	5.9	5.6	5.4	5.2	23.8
210	5.5	5.2	5.0	4.8	22.1
200	5.0	4.8	4.6	4.4	20.2
190	4.6	4.4	4.2	4.1	18.7
185	4.4	4.2	4.0	3.9	17.8
180	4.2	4.0	3.9	3.7	17.0
175	4.0	3.8	3.7	3.5	16.2
170	3.8	3.6	3.5	3.3	15.3
165	3.6	3.4	3.3	3.1	14.4
160	3.4	3.2	3.1	3.0	13.7
155	3.2	3.0	2.9	2.8	12.8
150	2.9	2.8	2.7	2.6	11.9
145	2.7	2.6	2.5	2.4	11.0
140	2.5	2.4	2.3	2.2	10.1
135	2.3	2.2	2.1	2.0	9.3
130	2.1	2.0	1.9	1.8	8.4

B: Less than 20-Pounds Overweight

Present Weight	Week 1	Week 2	Week 3	Week 4	Total Month (4.3 weeks)
200	3.5	3.4	3.2	3.1	14.2
190	3.3	3.2	3.0	2.9	13.4
185	3.2	3.1	3.0	2.9	13.2
180	3.2	3.1	2.9	2.8	12.9

Maximum Fat-Tissue Loss (72% Fat, 22% Water, 6% Protein)				
Present Weight	Week 1	Week 2	Week 3	Week 4	Total Month (4.3 weeks)
175	3.1	3.0	2.9	2.8	12.7
170	3.0	2.9	2.8	2.7	12.3
165	2.9	2.7	2.6	2.5	11.5
160	2.7	2.6	2.5	2.4	11.0
155	2.6	2.5	2.4	2.4	10.7
150	2.6	2.5	2.3	2.3	10.5
145	2.4	2.3	2.2	2.2	9.8
140	2.3	2.2	2.1	2.0	9.3
135	2.2	2.0	1.9	1.8	8.4
130	2.0	1.9	1.8	1.8	8.4
125	1.9	1.8	1.7	1.7	7.7
120	1.7	1.6	1.5	1.5	6.8
115	1.5	1.4	1.3	1.3	5.9
110	1.3	1.2	1.2	1.1	5.2

20-pounds-overweight barrier, she should use Section B to estimate her weight-loss for the next 4 weeks.

At the end of each 4-week period, she should be sure to switch to her new *actual* weight figure. In this example, she reached 136.8 pounds after 4 weeks, which was still more than 20-pounds overweight, so she still used Section A. At the end of the next 4-week period she was 128.2 pounds, which is less than 20-pounds overweight. Therefore, her next 4-week projection should come from Section B.

Note in Table 14-2 that the woman in the example lost a little more than 2 pounds a week, just about perfect. Her appearance improved after losing 10 pounds in only 4 weeks, going from "very fat" to "heavy" in only 6 weeks, and on to "acceptable" in a total of 9 weeks would be

TABLE 14-2–14-3
Example of Fat-Loss Progress

14-2: A Woman Weighing 147 Pounds and 32-Pounds Overweight

Diet Week	Figure Status	Start Weight	Table Section	Table Line	Weight Loss	Finish Weight	Total Loss
1	Very Fat	147.0	A	145	2.7	144.3	2.7
2		144.3	–	–	2.6	141.7	5.3
3		141.7	–	–	2.5	139.2	7.8
4	Fat	139.2	–	–	2.4	136.8	10.2
5		136.8	A	135	2.3	134.5	12.5
6	Heavy	134.5	–	–	2.2	132.3	14.7
7		132.3	–	–	2.1	130.2	16.8
8		130.2	–	–	2.0	128.2	18.8
9	Acceptable	128.2	B	130	2.0	126.2	20.8
10		126.2	–	–	1.9	124.3	22.7
11		124.3	–	–	1.8	122.5	24.5
12	Nice	122.5	–	–	1.8	120.7	26.3
13		120.7	B	120	1.7	119.0	28.0
14		119.0	–	–	1.6	117.4	29.6
15		117.4	–	–	1.5	115.9	31.1
15.5	Perfect	115.9	–	–	0.9	115.0	32.0

Average Rate of Loss: 2.1 pounds per week.

14-3: A Man Weighing 184 Pounds and 15-Pounds Overweight

Diet Week	Figure Status	Start Weight	Table Section	Table Line	Weight Loss	Finish Weight	Total Loss
1	Fat	184.0	B	185	3.2	180.8	3.2
2	Chunky	180.8	–	–	3.1	177.7	6.3
3	Acceptable	177.7	–	–	3.0	174.7	9.3
4	Good	174.7	–	–	2.9	171.8	12.2
5	Perfect	171.8	B	(170)	(2.8)	169.0	15.0

Average Rate of Loss: 3 pounds per week.

quite dramatic and would quickly renew her pride in herself.

Reducing from 32-pounds overweight in less than 16 weeks would allow time for the woman's appestat (hunger-control center) to reset itself, allow time for her new eating patterns to become permanent, and move her gradually to her ideal weight.

Table 14-3 illustrates the use of Table 14-1 in estimating the rate of fat-loss for a 184-pound man who is 15-pounds overweight. He will lose an average of 3 pounds a week, which is perfect for a man of his weight. It's easier for a man to lose fat, and as seen in this example, he could go from "fat" to "perfect weight" in just 5 weeks.

YOUR OWN FAT-LOSS PROGRAM CHART

How fast will you lose flab? Use Table 14-1 to predict. Construct your own Fat-Loss Program Chart as in the examples 14-2 and 14-3. Whether or not you follow the loss patterns of the average dieter used in the tables depends on several factors. It's almost certain you will fall into a grouping that's between 70 percent as fast as the average rate and 30 percent faster. If you are losing weight faster than this range (i.e., losing the same amount of weight in only two thirds of the time), you had better slow down by eating more food. Otherwise, you will be losing needed lean tissue. With success, you will have put on a pound or two of muscle to better support your figure.

It is permissible to lose more weight than charted during the first 2 weeks when you are also burning sugar stored in muscle and reducing your food bulk. Save your chart of estimated rate of fat-loss (Table 14-1) to compare with your actual rate of loss (Table 15-1) so that you won't go too fast.

LOSING WEIGHT TOO FAST

Let's look at what happens when you cut back too far on the amount of good food you eat. Let's assume that the average 145-pound person needs 2,175 calories of food energy to maintain that weight. For simplicity, we'll ignore food quality (and FLAB Units) to concentrate on body-energy needs. If that person goes on a 1,200-calorie diet, the body will have to make up the 975-calorie deficit by mobilizing its stored reserves and/or lean tissue.

The amount of fat that can be mobilized varies according to genetic factors and food quality, but let's assume this dieter can mobilize a quarter pound (actually this dieter could mobilize 0.27 pounds) of fat to provide the 975 calories of energy. This would amount to a loss in fat tissue of 0.39 pounds, because the water associated with the fat in the fat tissue would be liberated as the fat was mobilized. Thus, this average person would lose 2.7 pounds of fat tissue in a week of which 1.9 pounds were pure fat.

Now if this same 145-pound person were placed on a 600-calorie diet, the daily calorie deficit would be 1,575 calories. (The liquid predigested protein diet suggests 480 to 600 calories daily for women and that's really not enough.) Since the person in our example was already mobilizing fat at the maximum rate, to provide 975 calories, the additional 600 calories needed would be removed from lean tissue.

Here's the catch. Each calorie of lean tissue burned produces 4½ times the weight-loss of a calorie of fat tissue. (Lean tissue is 70 percent water, and water is heavy.) However, a pound of lean tissue provides only 563 calories.

The extra 600-calorie deficit will cause the person to lose 1.1 pounds of lean tissue, whereas the first 975-calorie deficit resulted in the loss of only 0.27 pounds of fat tissue.

TABLE 14-4
Estimating Your Desired Progress

Diet Week	Figure Status	Starting Weight	Table Section	Table Line	Weight Loss	Finish Weight	Total Loss
1							
2							
3							
4							
5							
6							
7							
8							

Dieters who judge their progress by the scale will be ecstatic at losing 1.37 pounds per day. That's 9.6 pounds per week compared to only 2.7 pounds on the Easy No-Flab Diet.

But when such dieters go off this very low-calorie diet, their bodies will try to regain the needed lean tissue and their weight will rebound as quickly as it fell off.

It can only be hoped that this will happen before serious health effects occur from the loss of lean tissue.

If you learn to appreciate the importance of keeping your health and losing only fat, you may develop greater patience in going about dieting the right way—surely and slowly. The Easy No-Flab Diet is perfectly safe and allows you to eat well and feel well as you selectively shed fat.

MEASURING YOUR FAT-LOSS

KEEPING A RECORD OF YOUR PROGRESS will see you through the emotional ups and downs when the scale seems stuck in one place or even goes the wrong way. And it will see you through times when you can't see any difference in your figure when you look in the mirror.

KEEPING AN ACCURATE RECORD

An accurate record will also warn you if you're losing weight too fast. Your first step is to prepare to keep such a record by making a projection of your anticipated weekly fat-loss, using Table 14-4. Your next step is to plot your actual results in terms of weight-loss, inches lost, and skin-fold thinning.

Figure 15-1 is a convenient chart for keeping track of your progress. To prepare your chart, write in your present weight at point A near the top on the left-hand side of the chart. Then write the pounds in descending order down the left-hand column. Note that the total pounds lost are already marked in the right-hand column.

FIGURE 15-1

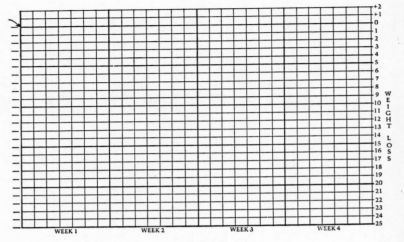

Weight-Loss Progress Chart

The first step in charting your progress is to construct a curve on the chart indicating the projected fat-loss for the average person at your present weight. To do this, first transfer the figures for your calculated pounds of fat-loss by the end of each week from Table 14-4 to Figure 15-1. Do this by placing an "X" on each heavy black vertical line (which represents the end of a week). Do it where the line intersects with that week's projected loss. Next, draw a smooth line through all of the "Xs." Starting at Point A. Remember, this line indicates the projected fat-loss for an average person, not necessarily for you. Charting your progress is the second step.

Two simple steps will help you keep track of your fat-loss progress. First, enter your current weight at Point A. Then list pounds in descending order down the left-hand column. Next mark with an "X" the intersections of your projected weekly losses on the heavy lines at the end of each week. Now draw a smooth curved line through all of the "Xs."

The second step is to record your actual weight each morning by placing an "X" at the appropriate point on the chart.

You can record progressive 4-week cycles on this one chart because your weight will continue to drop.

Each morning, after answering nature's call, record your weight on the chart where the figure for your weight intersects with the line for that day. You can readily see if your progress is following the projected line within reasonable limits (which would be between 70 percent slower and/or 30 percent faster than the rate indicated by the line). It's okay to exceed this rate for the first 2 weeks.

But don't put all your emphasis on the weight-loss chart. Your actual weight-loss will be irregular with all kinds of ups and downs. The chart is of value only over the long haul—not week to week.

Figure 15-2 compares the projected curve for the 184-pound man who was 15-pounds overweight to supposed day-to-day variations obtained for the sake of example.

YOUR FIRST 2 WEEKS ON THE DIET

Possibly a dieter's greatest mistake comes in misinterpreting any initial rapid weight-loss as something that can be continued at nearly the same rate. While this initial rapid loss, if it occurs, may be encouraging and does the ego good, it can have the smashing effect of severe discouragement later. Many times dieters have had the first 2 pounds fall right off. But when their weight then fluctuated up and down a bit, they often become angry or disillusioned. They may then have gone off the diet and on an eating binge.

FIGURE 15-2

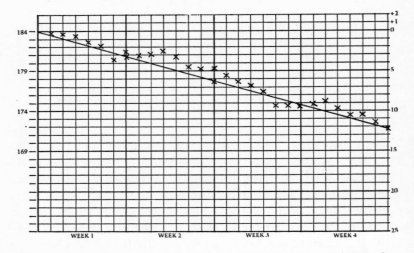

Comparison of "Actual" Progress Against Projected Weight-Loss for a 184-Pound Man.

An extra-fast initial weight-loss sometimes comes about because of reduced food bulk and extra water-loss. This is a weight-loss, but not flab-loss. Don't be discouraged if you don't lose the same number of pounds per day during the second week. Be encouraged that much of your weight-loss that week will have been flab-loss.

Some dieters may not have that initial rapid loss, because their systems turn around more slowly. They may not lose any weight for 3 days, then progress smoothly.

MEASURING INCHES LOST

Now let's get the tape measure and fill in Table 15-3. Measure your waist at its smallest circumference, take other measurements at the largest circumferences. Be

TABLE 15-3
Inches-Off Progress Chart

Diet Week	Waist	Hips	Thighs	Calves	Chest/ Bust	Upper Arm
1						
2						
3						
4						
5						
6						
7						
8						

sure to keep the tape in a straight line along this circumference, perpendicular to the length of the limb or trunk. (Often when people try to take their own measurements, they measure on a slant, which gives an inaccurate reading.) Keep the tape snug, but not tight. The tape should *measure* the circumference, not shorten it.

During the periods when your scale weight seems unchanged primarily due to water-retention fluctuations, it will be reassuring to refer to the inches-off progress chart.

At times your weight will decrease slowly, because as fat is being burned off, new muscle or lean tissue will be formed. If you have lost a pound of fat, but gained a pound of muscle, the scale will show no difference, but the tape measure will. Muscle tissue is denser so a pound of muscle will take up less space than a pound of fat.

As you monitor your inches lost, you will usually find that the loss in various areas of your body is not proportional. First one area will show more loss than another, then vice versa.

The areas where you lose fat tissue first will be determined mostly by your family characteristics.

If your family looks "hippy," then you can be reasonably sure fat will go to your hips first and come off your hips last. But fat will come off your hips continually, and you will not get overly skinny everywhere else first.

"Spot" reducing or "spot" exercising will not change your rate of fat-loss in any area. "Spot" exercises will, however, help shape that area, so they're a good idea.

Have faith that all of your flab will come off without destroying your curves. It's only a matter of time as long as you stick with the diet—and it's easy to stick with the Easy No-Flab Diet.

MEASURING SKIN-FOLD PROGRESS

In Chapter 13 you learned how to measure your fat accurately by taking skin-fold measurements. Record your progress in Table 15-4.

THE TOTAL PICTURE OF YOUR PROGRESS

Table 15-5 will give you a capsule overview of your progress. A mirror will indicate your present figure status, but don't trust your memory to judge your progress. You may not notice your day-by-day improvement, but photographs will jog your memory. Have several full-length photographs taken before you begin the diet. For the photos, stand relaxed in a tight-fitting bathing suit near an uncluttered wall. You should have front, side, and back views taken as shown in Figure 15-6.

TABLE 15-4
Record of Skin-fold Measurements

Diet Week	Triceps	Biceps	Back	Waist	TOTAL
1					
2					
3					
4					
5					
6					
7					
8					

TABLE 15-5
Summary of Major Indicators

Diet Week	Weight	Waist Measurement	Waist Skin fold	Hip Measurement	Triceps Skin fold	Fit of Clothing	Figure Status
1							
2							
3							
4							
5							
6							
7							
8							

FIGURE 15-6
Pictures Don't Lie

Pictures do not lie. Don't underestimate the value of full-length photos as aids in comparing your progress. Stand relaxed near an uncluttered wall, and have front, side, and back views taken. You may not notice your gradual day-by-day progress, but these photos will jog your memory.

EXERCISE WILL SPEED YOUR FAT-LOSS

Keep in mind that your shape *is* changing. It's common for women to drop from size 12 to size 8, even while gaining a few pounds—if they exercise. Without exercise, you will lose the flab, but you will not get rid of all the fat within the muscles that gives muscles the marbled look of good-tasting, but fatty beef.

The Easy No-Flab Program includes exercises to "clean" your lean tissue of fat, shape you, and speed your rate of flab-loss. Without the proper exercise you can slim down, but you will still have a fat shape. A little exercise will reshape you and make you slender, slinky, and make your body function better. Don't skip the next chapter. It will tell you why exercise is so important in speeding up your fat-loss.

SPEEDING UP YOUR FAT-LOSS

YOU CAN SPEED UP THE RATE AT WHICH you burn fat in three ways. All three involve stepping up your level of activity. The easiest way to do this is with a pleasant exercise program involving striding, interval jogging, or swimming—whichever you prefer. Just 30 minutes 3 times a week or 20 minutes 5 times a week is all you'll need.

REGULAR EXERCISE SPEEDS FAT-LOSS

Regular exercise has a hidden benefit. It does more than just burn calories while you are exercising; it steps up basal metabolism (calories burned while resting). With a stepped-up metabolism, you burn more calories even when you're resting. This effect is barely noticeable in women. Again, it's easier for men to lose weight.

Occasional exercise does not increase metabolic rate, only regular exercise in which the heart and lungs must work at near 70 to 80 percent of capacity for a period of 20 minutes or more. You don't have to exercise constantly during that period, as long as you don't rest so long that your pulse and respiration fall below 70 percent of your capacity. This is the principle behind interval training (that's exercising at 70 to 80 percent of capacity and resting alternately). Interval training, which can be applied to swimming, running, or striding is discussed further in Appendix II.

A person appreciably overweight can lose flab readily without exercising, but a person only 5- to 10-pounds overweight has a lower percentage of fat stored as flab beneath the skin. Thus the person only slightly overweight has more difficulty in burning fat at an appreciable rate, without exercising to burn the marbleized fat within the muscles.

All people should exercise in some form. If you don't use your body—you'll lose it. Unfortunately the only exercise many people get is exercising their resistance to exercise. But no matter how much we are out of shape, there is a moderate, progressive way back to proper body function.

THE DIETER'S FIRST EXERCISE—THE "PUSH-BACK"

Dieters particularly need to exercise. First of all, they must learn the "push-back," that's pushing away from the table when they've eaten the right amount of good food.

What's on the table is on the lips for only a second, but it may stay on the hips forever if you don't exercise the "push-back."

STRONGER MUSCLES BURN MORE FAT

A side benefit of exercise is that stronger muscles burn more fat all day long, even when you're resting or sleeping. Consistent exercise increases the amount of the fat-burning enzymes in the muscles.

An important factor in developing more of the fat-burning enzymes is the length of time you spend exercising. It's possible to exercise too hard and lose lean tissue because of muscle damage. So, therefore, exercise longer, not harder. **A long walk every day is better than a fast run once in a while.**

If you exercise daily, you need only 12 minutes. If you exercise 5 days a week, you need 20 minutes daily. If you exercise 3 times a week, you need to exercise 30 minutes each time

It is true that the more vigorous the activity, the more calories will be burned in the same amount of *time*. However, the *amount* of work you do will determine the energy you'll need. **Striding a mile in 15 minutes burns essentially the same amount of fat as jogging or running a mile in half that time.** There is a slight difference in that joggers do more work because they raise their feet higher.

By the way, don't let those tables in Chapter 26 that list the calories expended in various activities discourage you. They are probably underestimates. What you need to know is that the more work you do, the more fat you will burn.

LACK OF EXERCISE IS THE MAIN CAUSE OF OBESITY

The reason that most people put on flab is not that they eat more but that they exercise less. The double-barrelled blast of expending fewer calories in activity and slowing metabolism, while still eating the same out of habit, is the main cause of obesity.

Trying to correct the situation by cutting down on food intake alone will lead to a state of constant dieting, during which the risk of inadequate nutrient intake is very great. Also your weight may move up and down like a roller coaster.

Some fat people really do eat less than most skinny people, but their activity level is too low, and they have developed the fat-storing body chemistry.

IT'S THOSE LITTLE THINGS THAT PUT WEIGHT ON AND TAKE IT OFF

It's the little things that accumulate a calorie at a time that put fat on. Maybe it's one less trip up the stairs each day, or another half hour sitting at the office instead of puttering around the yard.

A woman would need to eat an average of only 96 calories a day more than she expends to gain 50 pounds in 5 years. If she also adds 25 minutes of brisk walking to her daily activities, this weight-gain would never occur.

The best way to burn the fat is in a pleasant, moderate exercise program until you reach your desired weight. If you can't exercise naturally in routine daily home activities (house cleaning/maintenance and yard work), you will have to continue the exercise program to maintain your desired weight. But, if you resume your life-style with the same zest you had before you started putting on the fat, you will stay naturally slender.

STARTING YOUR DIET

YOU'RE NOW READY, BETTER YET, EAGER to start the Easy No-Flab Diet. But if you do start without the proper preparation, you'll increase your risk of quitting the diet on the spur of the moment. Really, there's little to prepare for, but what there is, is important.

Fortunately, there's no need to steel yourself for self-denial. Just relax and decide now to do it right, right from the start. No diet is sheer delight, but it doesn't have to be drudgery either.

Proper planning and the right frame of mind go a long way in successful dieting. The Easy No-Flab Diet will allow you to take control of your body chemistry and make you naturally slender without hunger or aggravation—provided you take the following preparation steps.

GIVE YOUR DOCTOR A PHONE CALL

Before you start the diet, call your physician and explain that you want to begin a new diet program. Tell your doctor that the Easy No-Flab Diet is a balanced diet of high-quality, low-insulin-release foods, having 1,200 calories (for women; for men, it's closer to 1,500). Explain that the daily diet is approximately 35 percent protein, 35 percent carbohydrate and 30 percent fat—that it contains about 105 gm of protein, about 105 gm of carbohydrate, mostly complex carbohydrate, and 40 gm of fat. Then read a few sample menus, so your doctor can judge the quality of the food you'll be enjoying.

Ask your physician if you have any medical conditions that make it inadvisable for you to use this diet. Are you taking any medication that would be interfered with by the foods in the diet? Are you allergic to any? Does your doctor feel this is a good time for you to diet? Ask if you should go in for a checkup before starting the diet.

GET YOUR "TOOLS" TOGETHER

After getting your doctor's approval, round up a measuring cup, measuring spoons, and a diet scale (a postage scale is okay). You'll also need a notebook to record your food intake for the next 3 days. When you note how many calories you've been eating you'll understand why your weight isn't where you want it to be. And the notebook will also help you see when you eat from hunger and when you eat from habit or social purpose. Keep your record on a chart similar to Figure 15-1 (see Figure 17-1).

You'll also need high-quality vitamin and mineral supplements as discussed in Chapter 24.

The vitamin and mineral supplements are required because although your food quantity will be restricted, you'll still need the same number of nutrients as always. And because the extra physical and mental stress imposed by dieting will consume more nutrients, you'll need to replace these to maintain your health.

You will be drinking either 4-, 6-, or 8-fluid ounces of various beverages, so you may find it advantageous to

119

FIGURE 17-1
Daily Food Chart

Fill out the chart for 3 days before starting the diet.
List all food you eat each day—including all your snacks.

TIME	FOOD	HUNGER HABIT OR SOCIAL	MOOD	PLACE	ACTIVITY	DID YOU FEEL FOOD WAS NECESSARY?	QUANTITY	CALORIES

find glasses that contain those amounts while appearing full (a psychological ploy) and yet not spilling. As an example, you'll do better drinking your 6-oz beverages from an 8-oz glass than from either a 6-oz capacity glass, which would invite spillage, or from a 12-oz glass, which would look too empty. The empty-looking glass will either make you feel like you're punishing yourself by doing without, or it will tempt you to pour in just a little bit more.

START THE 3-DAY DIET WARM-UP

It will take 3 days to get ready for the Easy No-Flab Diet Program. Continue eating as you normally do while keeping your food-intake record.

> On day one of this warm-up period, be sure to drink an 8-fluid-ounce glass of cool water or water with a teaspoon or tablespoon of lemon juice or unsweetened lemonade in it at midmorning, and again about 2 hours after dinner. Continue this every day during the next 2 warm-up days and all during the diet. You'll probably find yourself looking forward to it.

> On day two of your preparation, eat 1 slice of cheese with each glass of water.

> On day three, make a conscious effort to cut down on eating candy, cookies, cake, and other sweets, and proceed as on day two.

GET YOUR ENVIRONMENT READY

During your 3-day preparation for the diet, get rid of the junk food in your living environment. Even gorge yourself one last time *if you must.*

Prepare yourself mentally by thinking how proud you'll be of your naturally slender body in just 6 or 8 weeks.

Remove magazines, free food coupons, or anything else that will tempt you to break the diet.

Now look at the first week's diet menu and buy only those foods, or the foods you may substitute for them. The flexibility of the diet is discussed in the following chapter. You have the option of substituting one meat for another or one vegetable for another, using FLAB Units as a guide.

Buy only items you need for the diet and leave the store. Above all, don't go to the grocery store on an empty stomach.

Check off This List Before Starting Your Diet

The diet preparation is just as important as the diet itself. Don't start until you have:
- ☐ Doctor's permission.
- ☐ Removed junk food.
- ☐ Removed food temptations.
- ☐ Had 2 8-oz glasses of water 3 days in a row.
- ☐ Had a slice of cheese with each glass of water 2 days in a row.
- ☐ Cut back on sweets on day three.
- ☐ Started taking a vitamin/mineral supplement.

THE EASY NO-FLAB DIET PROGRAM

18 NO ONE WANTS TO WORK AT LOSING FAT all day long. But if your body isn't primed to burn stored fat all day long, you have a slim chance of losing your fat. The trick is to set your body up for burning fat and keeping it stoked-up 24 hours a day without much conscious effort.

On the Easy No-Flab Diet, you won't feel as though you're dieting because you won't be hungry—and you'll be eating well, and often. Still, you won't be able to make exceptions in the program by eating poor foods, more FLAB Units, or skipping some of the good food, because that would shut down your fat-burning mechanism.

You will have to eat full meals and snacks. You won't have to "work" at dieting all day long, unless you consider eating good food to be work. Maybe it will seem like work at first, but you'll soon realize that good food is good-tasting and you'll begin to look forward to your meals. It's imperative that you do your morning sit-ups and exercise about a half hour 3 times a week or 12 minutes 5 times a week.

IT'S FLEXIBLE

The program is flexible. You can either follow the suggested menus, or devise your own as long as your meals meet a few basic requirements. If you follow the suggested menus, you don't have to be concerned about counting FLABs—or calories, or protein, or carbohydrate, or anything else. Just follow the menus exactly.

After a few meals, you'll learn portion sizes for most foods, without measuring cups. As examples, a half cup of orange juice or three quarters' cup of milk can be accurately estimated by using the designs on the glasses as guides. However, I do suggest you weigh your meats each time after cooking.

A FEW GUIDELINES

The only rules you will have to remember are:

1. Never skip a meal.
2. Eat *all* the food in the meals and snacks.
3. Don't skip a snack during the first 2 weeks. Later you can cut back on snacks, but you must still drink the water.
4. Do 10 sit-ups as soon as you can after waking up each morning.
5. Exercise for about 30 minutes 3 times a week or for 12 minutes 5 times a week.
6. Do not eat foods not included in the suggested menus or those you have designed yourself according to the following rules.

DESIGNING YOUR OWN MENUS

If you design your own menus, you will have to remember some additional rules:

1. Women should eat between 900 and 1,100 FLABs daily, while men should eat between 1,000 and 1,300.
2. Include at least 60 gm, but preferably 100 gm, of protein daily.
3. Don't eat foods ranking below 50 on the FLAB Index.
4. Design your meals to average about 335 FLABs.
5. Drink 6 glasses of water each day. That's a glass at each meal and a glass at each snack.
6. Make sure you get plenty of fiber and B-Complex vitamins to prevent constipation.
7. Eat 3 snacks during the first 7 to 10 days. After that you may taper off the snacks for convenience or to adjust weight loss.

The choice is yours: you can follow the suggested menus, all, or as many as you like—or design your own.

A TYPICAL DAY ON THE DIET

On your first day of the diet, after your 3 days' preparation, you should stick to the following schedule (Table 18-1). It's the schedule you should follow every day you're on the diet. In just a few days the eight steps on the schedule will become a pleasant routine.

Just eight steps during 14 hours shouldn't be that hard especially when after about a week you'll actually enjoy the good feeling that comes from the exercise and from meals filled with a great variety of good foods. Note the foods in Table 18-2 that can wreck your program, and avoid them.

How good are the menus? Well, you can look for yourself in the next 3 chapters.

TABLE 18-1
Daily Activity

Time	Activity
After waking up (can be done in bed)	10 sit-ups
Breakfast	No-Flab Breakfast of your choice Supplements
Midmorning	Snack (water plus cheese or egg)
Lunch	No-Flab Lunch of your choice
Midafternoon	Snack (water plus cheese or egg)
Dinner	No-Flab Dinner of your choice Supplements
Midevening	Exercise Period 30 minutes 3 times/week OR 12 minutes 5 times/week
Before Retiring	Snack (water plus popcorn or celery)

TABLE 18-2
Foods That Will Wreck the Program

Foods having a FLAB Index rating of less than 50 will ruin your Easy No-Flab Diet Program. See Appendix III for a listing of FLAB Indexes for the foods eaten most often. The following are examples of foods you should avoid:

*Alcoholic Beverages
Cake
Candy
Cookies
Condensed Milk
†Honey
Jam
Jelly
Marmalade
Mineral Oil for salad dressing
Molasses
Pie
Preserves
Sugar

---

*Alcoholic beverages are a bad idea during the first 2 weeks of your diet because alcohol disrupts the blood-sugar level. Later, you can have 1 oz of wine, 6 oz of beer, or 1/2 oz of spirits any day, if you omit 75 FLABs of bread or starchy vegetable. If you get hungry, cut out the alcohol.

†One-half teaspoon of honey can be used with the Diet-Shake Program.

EASY NO-FLAB BREAKFASTS

19   "I DON'T HAVE TIME FOR BREAKFAST." "I can't eat breakfast." "If I eat breakfast too, I'll *really* be fat." Such are the comments I hear from overweight people. These same people usually explain that when they do eat breakfast, they feel bad. So, instead, they may opt for a cup of coffee and a cigarette.

The "no breakfast" people run into low blood-sugar problems (weakness, fatigue, loss of concentration) about 3 hours after waking up and either take a coffee break or smoke a cigarette. They don't realize that without breakfast their morning performance is not at its best. Nor do they realize that their eating pattern—one or two meals a day, with most of the calories coming after most of the day's activities—leads to fat deposits.

When these people shift to a substantial breakfast plus lunch and dinner, they are soon amazed at their increased energy and better proportioned figures. More of the potential energy in their food is used for their immediate needs (ready energy, not stored energy), because this potential energy is in the bloodstream when the body actually needs it.

It's when you eat after your body's immediate energy

needs have been met that the potential energy in the food is stored as fat.

The "no breakfast" people experience wild gyrations in their blood-sugar levels and that causes energy problems, emotional problems, and mental-acuity problems. The breakfast-skippers rely on nicotine and caffeine to give them pick-ups. Because they shoot their blood-sugar levels up with non-food stimulants, they shortchange their body's nutrient supply and so they are more susceptible to the entire range of diseases that attack the human body.

When they do sit down to eat, they overeat because their appetite control center (appestat) is malfunctioning and the energy from most of the food they eat is diverted to fat storage for tomorrow's needs. And so these people tend to have full fat cells.

THE BIG BREAKFAST

It is true that some people have trouble shifting to a large breakfast, but slowly increasing the size of their breakfast will overcome the problems.

Studies also show that students do better with good breakfasts. One of the reasons is that their blood sugar remains level and they are able to concentrate better.

More than 20 years ago, the Iowa Breakfast Studies showed that people getting at least an ounce (28.4 gm) of protein for breakfast performed their tasks, at work or school, better than those who ate less than an ounce of protein for breakfast.

All the Easy No-Flab Diet Breakfasts contain at least an ounce of protein, with the typical breakfast having an ounce and a quarter (35 gm).

The Iowa Breakfast Studies also found that protein at breakfast stabilized the blood-sugar levels for long periods. Even if plenty of protein is eaten later in the day to more than satisfy the daily requirements, it is too late to compensate for the missed morning protein needs. The heavier protein feeding later in the day cannot smooth out the gyrating blood-sugar level as well as the same amount distributed more evenly, when needed. Also, there may be more protein than the body can use when the larger quantity of protein is eaten in a single meal, and this is wasted because it is converted to fat. The timing in eating protein is as important as the quantity.

People who miss a meal or eat less nutrients than they need become hungry, irritable, jumpy, and anxious. A hearty breakfast protects against this.

THE DANGER PERIODS

Dieters on less-than-perfect diets often lose their willpower because of these symptoms. The three danger periods for a dieter are midmorning, late-afternoon, and bedtime. A proper breakfast will control the midmorning and many of the late-afternoon problems, by stabilizing the blood-sugar level to prevent hunger and fat storage.

TIME FOR BREAKFAST

If you "don't have time" for breakfast, consider the 5-minute blender meals or the Diet Shakes described in Chapter 23, or just get up a half hour earlier. The blender breakfasts typically are eggs and fruit blended with milk, and the Diet Shakes are protein powder plus fruit or flavoring blended with milk or juice. They can be prepared the night before by blending at top speed for a full minute (or vigorous hand shaking). If desired, they can be stored overnight in the refrigerator with a 10-second refresher blend or shake in the morning.

You can even save time in the morning with regular breakfasts by setting everything up before going to bed the night before.

THE DISASTER BREAKFAST

The typical diet suggests a bare-bones breakfast because most people don't get really hungry until they move around for a while in the morning. During sleep your body has been rebuilding its blood-sugar level.

Most diets shave calories at breakfast because of the absence of "deep" hunger and the fact that many people are not fully awake at the breakfast table and are still too tired to eat. Most diets suggest a low-calorie, high-carbohydrate breakfast. This is disastrous. This will start the blood-sugar level in a tizzy that results in hunger and fatigue at midmorning.

Even the high-protein diets usually stress low-calorie breakfasts, and this is disastrous because you need a full third of the day's energy at breakfast.

On a reducing diet, you should get about 320 to 360 FLAB Units at breakfast. Ideally, this is equal to about 375 to 400 calories, consisting of approximately 35 gm of protein, 35 gm of carbohydrate (mostly complex) and 13 gm of fat.

The predominantly carbohydrate breakfast may be filling while you are eating, but an hour or so later you will be starving. The fat is needed for flavor, satiety, and long-term energy, and the protein for body repair and medium-term energy.

Let's look at the different nutrient values of the Easy No-Flab Diet Breakfast and other breakfasts.

TABLE 19-1–19-2

19-1

No-Flab Breakfast	Quantity	Prote	Carbo	Fat	Vit A
Orange juice	4 oz	0.9	13.3	0.1	249
Skim milk	6 oz	5.5	8.4	0.2	375
Bread, whole wheat	1 sl	2.4	10.8	0.7	tr*
Egg	1 lrg	6.9	0.2	8.6	710
Ham, low-nitrite	2 oz	17.1	0	5.1	0
		32.8	32.7	14.7	1334
Typical Pancake Breakfast					
Hot cakes	3	5.7	26.4	6.0	204
Butter	1 tsp	tr	tr	4.1	165
Syrup	2 tsp	0.0	10.2	0.0	0
Coffee	3/4 cup	0.0	0.0	0.0	0
Sugar	1 tsp	0.0	3.4	0.0	0
		5.7	40.0	10.1	369
Typical Cereal Breakfast					
Skim milk	3/4 cup	5.5	8.4	0.2	375
Cereal	3/4 cup	1.5	16.0	0.1	0
Banana	1 med	1.3	26.4	0.2	226
Toast	1 sl	2.9	11.5	0.7	tr
Jelly	1 tbsp	0.0	12.2	0.0	2
Coffee, black	3/4 cup	0.0	0.0	0.0	0
		11.2	74.5	1.2	603

19-2

Breakfast Comparisons				
No-Flab	32.8	32.7	14.7	1334
Pancake	5.7	40.0	10.1	369
Cereal	12.2	74.5	1.2	603

*tr-trace (present, but too small to measure).

Vit C	Vit B_1	Vit B_2	Vit B_3	Ca	Iron	Vit D	Cals
56	0.11	0.01	0.40	11	0.10	00	56
3	0.08	0.36	0.16	228	0.08	750	58
tr	0.06	0.03	0.60	22.0	0.50	00	55
0	0.05	0.15	0.10	30.0	1.20	00	108
0	0.36	0.16	3.26	7.3	2.12	00	119
59	0.66	0.71	4.52	298.3	4.00	750	396
tr	0.18	0.24	0.9	174	0.9	0	183
0	0.00	0.00	0.0	0	0.0	0	36
0	0.00	0.00	0.0	0	0.0	0	42
0	0.00	0.00	0.5	3	0.2	0	2
0	0.00	0.00	0.0	0	0.0	0	14
tr	0.18	0.24	1.4	177	1.1	0	277
3	0.08	0.36	0.16	228	0.08	75	58
0	0.08	0.02	0.40	3	0.30	00	72
12	.06	.07	0.80	10	0.80	00	101
tr	.09	.06	0.80	19	0.60	00	61
1	tr	.01	0.00	4	0.30	00	49
0	0.00	0.00	0.50	3	0.20	00	2
16	0.31	.52	2.7	267	2.3	75	343
59	0.66	0.71	4.52	298	4.0	75	396
tr	0.18	0.24	1.4	177	1.1	0	277
16	0.31	0.52	2.7	267	2.3	75	343

PLANNING A TASTY BREAKFAST

The most satisfying way to achieve a nutritious breakfast balance is to plan a meal with:

Fruit	(either 1/2 cup juice or portion of whole fruit)
Skim milk	3/4 cup
Grain	1 slice of whole grain bread or 1 oz of cereal or 1 pancake (whole wheat or rye are excellent bread selections)
Protein	3 to 5 oz of meat, eggs, or cheese

The first food in the Easy No-Flab Diet Breakfast is from the fruit group.

One-half cup (4 fluid ounces) of orange juice contains 0.9 gm of protein, 13.3 gm of carbohydrates, and 0.1 gm of fat, and yields 57 FLAB Units.

The following foods may be substituted for the half cup of orange juice.

TABLE 19-3

Food	Quantity	FLABs	Prote (gm)	Carbo (gm)	Fat (gm)	Cals
Orange Juice	1/2 cup	57	0.9	13.3	0.1	58
Tomato	1/2 cup	25	1.1	5.2	0.1	26
Orange	1/3 med.*	24	0.5	5.5	0.1	32
Grapefruit	1/4 med.	24	0.3	6.3	0.1	24
Cantaloupe	1/4 med.	29	0.7	7.2	0.1	29

*A whole fruit is easily divided into thirds by first cutting it in half and then cutting each half into three equal slices. Two of the resulting six sections equal a third of the whole.

The second food in the Easy No-Flab Diet Breakfast is from the milk group. Normally 3/4 cup (6 fluid ounces) of skim milk will add protein, calcium, and fluid to your meal. Men may add 1 teaspoon of butter to their breakfast menu in addition to the milk.

If you are one of the 30 million Americans who has lactose intolerance, or is allergic to milk, drink water and add one teaspoon of butter to your meal to increase the calories. Of special interest to those with lactose intolerance are the digestive aides that can be purchased at health food stores to overcome the problem and allow them to drink the skim milk.

The third food in the Easy No-Flab Diet Breakfast is from the grain group. A slice of whole wheat bread contains 2.4 gm of protein, 10.8 gm of carbohydrate and 0.7

TABLE 19-4

Food	Quantity	FLABs	Prote (gm)	Carbo (gm)	Fat (gm)	Cals
Whole wheat bread	1 sl	51	2.4	10.8	0.7	55
Potatoes, hash brown	1 oz	51	1.2	10.2	0.7	52
Pancake whole wheat	4″	59	1.9	8.8	2.0	61
Oatmeal	1/2 cup	64	2.4	11.6	1.2	66
Bran flakes	2/3 cup	73	2.0	15.3	0.7	76
Corn flakes	2/3 cup	62	1.3	14.2	0.1	64
Wheat flakes	2/3 cup	60	1.9	13.5	0.1	65
Banana	1/2 med.	56	0.7	13.2	0.1	51
Corn bread	1 oz	61	2.0	9.8	1.7	63
Rye bread	1 sl	51	2.0	1.8	0.2	55
Hominy grits	1/2 cup	59	1.5	13.5	0.1	62
Waffle, whole wheat	1	61	2.1	8.1	2.5	65

gm of fat, yielding 51 FLAB Units. The following foods can be substituted for the slice of whole wheat bread.

The major portion of the required 28 gm of protein should come from a combination of two of three sources—eggs, meat, or cheese. The fruit, milk, and grain groups provide only 6 to 8 gm of the needed protein, so the protein group must provide 22 to 27 gm of protein. The following list provides excellent selections:

Coffee or tea (including iced tea and herbal teas) can be added to breakfast for those people accustomed to caffeine. Although caffeine disrupts the blood-sugar control and should be avoided, you should not attempt to break your caffeine habit while dieting. It's too much of a stress.

VARIETY IS THE SPICE OF LIFE

Several suggested breakfasts follow, but you are not limited to them. Have fun making up your own menus. Just be sure to keep the FLAB Units between 320 and 360, and to have at least 28 gm of protein in your breakfast. Breakfast like a king.

For economy, if a breakfast calls for a half cup of yogurt or half of a fruit, pick a lunch or dinner in which you can eat the rest, or share the rest with the family or friends. Even if you don't use the rest, it's cheaper to throw the excess away than to buy a larger wardrobe.

You should not have the same breakfast every day. You can rotate a minimum of four breakfast menus. Use your diet to sample different menus. Variety is the spice of life.

The breakfasts are independent of the lunch and dinner menus. You may choose any lunch or dinner to go with any breakfast, so nearly an endless combination of menus is possible. Enjoy them.

TABLE 19-5

Food	Quantity	FLABs	Prote (gm)	Carbo (gm)	Fat (gm)	Cals
Egg, fried	1 lrg	92	6.9	0.2	8.6	108
Egg, boiled	1 lrg	67	6.5	0.5	5.8	82
Egg, scrambled	1 lrg	95	7.2	1.5	8.3	111
Fish sticks with lemon juice	1 oz	52	5.4	1.9	3.8	64
Tuna	2 oz	74	16.4	0.0	4.6	112
Ham, low nitrite	1 oz	40	8.6	0.0	2.6	60
Cheese, cottage	2 oz	44	7.7	1.7	2.4	60
Cheese, American	1 sl	92	6.0	1.6	8.2	104
Muenster	1 oz	91	6.2	0.6	8.5	102
Sardines	1/2 of 3-3/4 oz can	92	11.0	0.0	8.0	115

Easy No-Flab Breakfast 1

Foods	Quantity	FLABs (gm)	Prote (gm)	Carbo (gm)	Fat (gm)	Cals
Orange juice	1/2 cup	57	0.9	13.3	0.1	58
Skim milk	6 oz 3/4 cup	46	5.5	8.4	.2	58
Bread, whole wheat	1 sl	51	2.4	10.8	0.7	55
Egg, fried	1 lrg	92	6.9	0.2	8.6	108
Ham (smoked or nitrite-free)	2 oz	80	17.1	0.0	5.1	119
Water	1 cup	0	0.0	0.0	0.0	0
		326	32.8	32.7	14.7	398

RECIPES

FRIED EGG

Heat 1 to 2 tablespoons butter in skillet until just hot enough to sizzle a drop of water. If you use a very large skillet, you will need more butter. Break and slip an egg into skillet. Reduce heat immediately. Cook slowly to desired degree of doneness, spooning butter over egg to baste, or turning egg to cook both sides. Makes 1 serving.

STEAM-BASTED VARIATION

Use just enough butter to grease skillet. Heat skillet until hot enough to sizzle a drop of water. Break and slip an egg into skillet. Cook over low heat until edges turn white, about 1 minute. Add 1 teaspoon water, decreasing proportion slightly for each additional egg being fried. Cover skillet tightly to hold in steam, which bastes the egg. Cook to desired degree of doneness. Makes 1 serving.

Easy No-Flab Breakfast 2

Food	Quantity	FLABs	Prote (gm)	Carbo (gm)	Fat (gm)	Cals
Tomato juice	4 oz	25	1.1	5.2	0.1	26
Skim milk	6 oz	46	5.5	8.4	0.2	58
Bread, whole wheat or Rye	1 sl	51	2.4	10.8	0.7	55
Breaded fish or fish sticks with fresh lemon juice	3 oz	157	16.2	5.8	11.3	193
Cottage cheese	2 oz	44	7.7	1.7	2.4	60
Water	1 cup	0	0.0	0.0	0.0	0
		323	32.9	31.9	14.7	392

Easy No-Flab Breakfast 3

Food	Quantity	FLABs	Prote (gm)	Carbo (gm)	Fat (gm)	Cals
Orange juice	1/2 cup	57	0.9	13.3	0.1	58
Skim milk	3/4 cup	46	5.5	8.4	0.2	58
Pancake	2–4" dia.	118	3.8	17.6	4.0	122
Ham (smoked or nitrite free)	2 oz	80	17.2	0.0	5.2	120
Cottage cheese	1 oz	22	3.9	0.9	1.2	30
Water	1 cup	0	0.0	0.0	0.0	0
		323	31.3	40.2	10.7	388

Easy No-Flab Breakfast 4

Food	Quantity	FLABs	Prote (gm)	Carbo (gm)	Fat (gm)	Cals
Orange juice	1/2 cup	57	0.9	13.3	0.1	58
Skim milk	3/4 cup	46	5.5	8.4	0.2	58
Egg, fried	1 lrg	92	6.9	0.2	8.6	108
Oatmeal (with part of the above milk)	1/2 cup	64	2.4	11.6	1.2	66
Ham	2 oz	80	17.2	–	5.2	120
Water	1 cup	0	0.0	0.0	0.0	0
		339	32.9	33.5	15.3	410

Easy No-Flab Breakfast 5

Food	Quantity	FLABs	Prote (gm)	Carbo (gm)	Fat (gm)	Cals
Orange juice	4 oz	57	0.9	13.3	0.1	58
Skim milk	6 oz	46	5.5	8.4	0.2	58
Bread, whole Wheat or Rye	1 sl	51	2.4	10.8	0.7	55
Egg, scrambled	1 lrg	95	7.2	1.5	8.3	111
Water	1 cup	0	0.0	0.0	0.0	0
Tuna (or any broiled fish)	2 oz	74	16.4	0.0	4.6	112
		323	32.4	34.0	13.9	394

RECIPE

SCRAMBLED EGG
1 egg
1 tbsp milk
1/8 tsp salt
Dash pepper
1 tbsp butter

Beat egg, milk salt and pepper together with fork, mixing thoroughly for uniform yellow, or mixing slightly for white and yellow streaks. Heat butter in skillet (approximately 8-inch) over medium heat until just hot enough to sizzle a drop of water. Pour in egg mixture. As mixture begins to set, gently draw pancake turner completely across the bottom, forming large soft curds. Continue until egg is thickened, but do not stir constantly. Cook until egg is thickened throughout but still moist.* Makes 1 serving.

*It is better to remove scrambled egg from pan when it is slightly underdone; heat retained in egg completes the cooking.

Easy No-Flab Breakfast 6

Food	Quantity	FLABs	Prote (gm)	Carbo (gm)	Fat (gm)	Cals
Tomato juice	1/2 cup	25	1.1	5.2	0.1	26
Skim milk	1 cup	61	7.3	11.3	0.2	77
Yogurt	1/2 cup	103	4.6	21.0	1.1	113
Fish sticks (or any breaded fish) with lemon juice	3 oz	157	16.2	5.8	11.3	193
Water	1 cup	0	0.0	0.0	0.0	0
		346	29.2	43.3	12.7	409

Easy No-Flab Breakfast 7

Food	Quantity	FLABs	Prote (gm)	Carbo (gm)	Fat (gm)	Cals
Tomato juice	1/2 cup	25	1.1	5.2	0.1	26
Skim milk	3/4 cup	46	5.5	8.4	0.2	58
Bread, whole wheat or rye	2 sl	102	4.8	21.6	1.4	110
Sardines	1/2 of 3 3/4-oz can	92	11.0	0.0	8.0	115
Cheese, Cheddar	1 sl	99	6.9	0.6	9.2	113
Water	1 cup	0	0.0	0.0	0.0	0
		364	29.3	35.8	18.9	422

Easy No-Flab Breakfast 8

Food	Quantity	FLABs	Prote (gm)	Carbo (gm)	Fat (gm)	Cals
Orange juice	1/2 cup	57	0.9	13.3	0.1	58
Skim milk	3/4 oz	46	5.5	8.4	0.2	58
Hash brown potatoes	1 oz	51	1.2	10.2	0.7	52
Egg (poached, soft, or hard-boiled	2 lrg	134	13.0	1.0	11.6	164
Ham (smoked or nitrite-free)	1 oz	40	8.6	0.0	2.6	60
Water	1 cup	0	0.0	0.0	0.0	0
		328	29.2	32.9	15.2	392

Easy No-Flab Breakfast 9

Food	Quantity	FLABs	Prote (gm)	Carbo (gm)	Fat (gm)	Cals
Peaches, fresh or water-pac	1/2 cup	98	0.5	24.0	0.1	100
Skim milk	3/4 oz	46	5.5	8.4	0.2	58
Cottage cheese with paprika	8 oz (cup)	175	30.8	6.6	9.6	240
Water	1 cup	0	0.0	0.0	0.0	0
		319	36.8	39.0	9.9	398

RECIPES

POACHED EGG
Lightly oil a saucepan. Add enough water* to make 2 inches deep. Heat to boiling. Reduce heat to hold temperature at simmering. Break egg into sauce dish; then slip egg into water, holding dish close to water's surface. Simmer 3 to 5 minutes, depending on degree of doneness desired. When done, remove egg with slotted pancake turner or spoon; drain on paper towel and trim edges, if desired.

*Milk or broth may be used instead of water

SOFT-COOKED EGG
Put egg in saucepan and add enough tap water to come at least 1 inch above egg. Cover, bring rapidly just to boiling. Turn off heat; if necessary, remove pan from burner to prevent further boiling. Let stand in the hot water 1 to 14 minutes, depending on desired degree of doneness. Cool eggs promptly in cold water for several seconds to prevent further cooking and to make them easier to handle.

To serve: break shell through middle with a knife. With a teaspoon, scoop egg out of each half shell into individual serving dish. If egg cup is used, slice off large end of egg with knife and eat from shell.

HARD-COOKED EGGS
Put egg into saucepan and add enough tap water to come at least 1 inch above egg. Cover, bring rapidly just to boiling. Let stand in the hot water 15 minutes for large eggs—adjust time up or down by approximately 3 minutes for each size larger or smaller. Cool immediately and thoroughly in cold water—shells are easier to remove and it is less likely you will have a dark surface on yolks. To remove shell: crackle it by tapping gently all over. Roll egg between hands to loosen shell; then peel, starting at large end. Hold egg under running cold water or dip in bowl of water to help ease off shell.

143

Easy No-Flab Breakfast 10

Food	Quantity	FLABs	Prote (gm)	Carbo (gm)	Fat (gm)	Cals
Cantaloupe	1/2 med.	58	1.4	14.4	0.2	58
Skim milk	3/4 cup	46	5.5	8.4	0.2	58
Bran flakes	2/3 cup	73	2.0	5.3	0.7	76
Skim milk (extra skim milk)	1/2 cup	30	3.7	5.7	0.1	39
Cottage cheese	6 oz	132	23.1	5.1	7.2	180
Water	1 cup	0	0.0	0.0	0.0	0
		339	35.7	48.9	8.4	411

Easy No-Flab Breakfast 11

Food	Quantity	FLABs	Prote (gm)	Carbo (gm)	Fat (gm)	Cals
Tomato juice	1/2 cup	25	1.1	5.2	0.1	26
Whole wheat toast	1 sl	51	2.4	10.8	0.7	55
Cheddar cheese	1 oz	99	6.9	0.6	9.2	113
Eggs	2	134	13.0	1.0	11.6	164
Butter	1 tbsp	36	0.0	0.0	4.1	36
Chives	1/2 tbsp	1	0.0	0.3		2
Water	1 cup	0	0.0	0.0	0.0	0
		346	23.4	17.9	25.7	395

RECIPE

CHIVED CHEESE OMELET

Measure cheese before preparing omelet; set aside. Mix eggs, 1/8 cup of water, chives, salt and pepper with fork. Heat butter in 10-inch omelet pan or skillet until just hot enough to sizzle a drop of water. Pour in egg mixture. Mixture should set at edges at once. With pancake turner, carefully draw cooked portions at edges toward center, so uncooked portions flow to bottom. Tilt skillet as it is necessary to hasten flow of uncooked eggs. Slide pan rapidly back and forth over heat to keep mixture in motion and sliding freely. While top is still moist and creamy-looking, sprinkle half of cheese over half of omelet. With pancake turner fold in half or roll, turning out onto platter with a quick flip of the wrist. Sprinkle remaining cheese over top of omelet. Makes 1 serving.

Easy No-Flab Breakfast 12

Food	Quantity	FLABs	Prote (gm)	Carbo (gm)	Fat (gm)	Cals
Tomato juice	1/2 cup	25	1.1	5.2	0.1	26
Skim milk	3/4 cup	46	5.5	8.4	0.2	58
Scrambled eggs	2 lrg	190	14.4	3.0	16.6	222
Cottage cheese	3 oz	66	11.6	2.5	3.6	90
Water	1 cup	0	0.0	0.0	0.0	0
		327	32.6	9.1	20.5	396

Easy No-Flab Breakfast 13

Food	Quantity	FLABs	Prote (gm)	Carbo (gm)	Fat (gm)	Cals
Grapefruit	1/4 med.	24	0.3	6.3	0.1	24
Skim milk	3/4 cup	46	5.5	8.4	0.2	58
Bread, whole wheat, rye or oatmeal	1 sl	51	2.4	10.8	0.7	55
Yogurt	1/2 cup	103	4.6	21.0	1.1	113
Cottage cheese	5 oz	110	19.3	4.3	6.0	150
Water	1 cup	0	0.0	0.0	0.0	0
		334	32.1	50.8	8.1	400

Easy No-Flab Breakfast 14

Food	Quantity	FLABs	Prote (gm)	Carbo (gm)	Fat (gm)	Cals
Vegetable juice	1/2 cup	25	1.1	5.2	0.1	26
Cantaloupe or Melon	1/4	29	0.7	7.2	0.1	29
Skim milk	3/4 cup	46	5.5	8.4	0.2	58
Hash browns	1 1/2 oz	75	1.8	17.3	1.0	78
Steak	3 1/2 oz	146	29.0	0.0	9.8	212
Water	1 cup	0	0.0	0.0	0.0	0
		321	38.1	38.1	11.2	403

Easy No-Flab Breakfast 15

Food	Quantity	FLAB	Prote (gm)	Carbo (gm)	Fat (gm)	Cals
Tomato juice	1/2 cup	25	1.1	5.2	0.1	26
Skim milk	3/4 cup	46	5.5	8.4	0.2	58
Hash browns	1 oz	51	1.2	10.2	0.7	52
Egg, poached	1 lrg	67	6.5	0.5	5.8	82
Fish sticks or Breaded fish	3 oz	157	16.2	5.8	11.3	193
Water	1 cup	0	0.0	0.0	0.0	0
		346	30.5	30.1	18.1	411

Easy No-Flab Breakfast 16

Food	Quantity	FLABs	Prote (gm)	Carbo (gm)	Fat (gm)	Cals
Grapefruit	1/2	48	0.6	12.6	0.2	48
Milk	3/4 cup	46	5.5	8.4	0.2	58
Cheddar cheese	1 oz	99	6.9	0.6	9.2	113
Fish sticks or Breaded fish	3 oz	157	16.2	5.8	11.3	193
Water	1 cup	0	0.0	0.0	0.0	0
		350	29.2	27.4	20.9	412

Easy No-Flab Breakfast 17

Food	Quantity	FLABs	Prote (gm)	Carbo (gm)	Fat (gm)	Cals
Skim milk Oatmeal with some of the skim milk)	3/4 cup 1/2 cup	46 64	5.5 2.4	8.4 11.6	0.2 1.2	58 66
Eggs, fried	2 lrg	184	13.8	0.4	17.2	216
Ham (smoked or nitrite-free)	1 oz	40	8.6	0.0	2.6	60
Water	1 cup	0	0.0	0.0	0.0	0
		334	30.3	20.4	21.2	400

Easy No-Flab Breakfast 18

Food	Quantity	FLABs	Prote (gm)	Carbo (gm)	Fat (gm)	Cals
Orange juice	1/2 cup	57	0.9	13.3	0.1	58
Skim milk	3/4 cup	46	5.5	8.4	0.2	58
Hominy grits (with 1 tsp butter)	1/2 cup	59	1.5	13.5	0.1	62
Ham	2 oz	80	17.2	0.0	5.2	120
Egg, fried	1 lrg	92	16.9	0.2	8.6	108
Water	1 cup	0	0.0	0.0	0.0	0
		334	32.0	35.4	14.2	406

BREAKFAST BLENDER SHAKES

The following Blender Shakes can be made occasionally as time-savers. You can also use any of the Diet Shakes described in Chapter 23.

The ingredients can be mixed with an egg beater or shaken vigorously in a "shaker" or jar, but best taste is obtained by mixing in a blender at the fastest speed for 1 minute. They are even more appealing when blended with three to four ice cubes.

You can thicken the shakes by blending them the night before and storing overnight in the refrigerator. Of course, you should blend again for 10 to 15 seconds before drinking in the morning.

Easy No-Flab Breakfast 19

Food	Quantity	FLABs	Prote (gm)	Carbo (gm)	Fat (gm)	Cals
O. J. Blender Shake *Mix in blender*						
Orange juice	1 cup	114	1.8	26.6	0.2	116
Skim milk	1 cup	62	7.3	11.3	0.2	77
Protein powder	1 oz	57	28.4	0.0	0.0	114
Lecithin	1 tbsp	108	0.0	0.0	12.0	108
Blend 1 minute at fastest speed						
Water	1 cup	0	0.0	0.0	0.0	0
		324	37.5	37.9	12.4	415

Easy No-Flab Breakfast 20

Food	Quantity	FLABs	Prote (gm)	Carbo (gm)	Fat (gm)	Cals
Banana Blender Shake *Mix in Blender*						
Eggs	2 lrg	134	13.0	1.0	11.6	164
Skim milk	2 cups	124	14.6	22.6	0.4	154
Banana	1/2 med.	55	0.7	13.2	0.1	57
Blend 1 minute at fastest speed						
Whole wheat or Rye toast	1/2 sl	26	1.2	5.4	0.4	28
Water	1 cup	0	0.0	0.0	0.0	0
		339	29.5	42.2	12.5	403

Easy No-Flab Breakfast 21

Foods	Quantity	FLABs	Prote (gm)	Carbo (gm)	Fat (gm)	Cals
EYE OPENER Blender Shake *Mix in Blender*						
Tomato Juice	1 cup	50	2.2	10.4	0.2	52
Eggs	2 lrg	134	13.0	1.0	11.6	164
Worcestershire sauce	1/8 tsp	0	0.0	tr*	0.0	0
Tobasco sauce	dash	3	0.0	1.0	0.0	3
Salt	pinch	0	0.0	0.0	0.0	0
Whole wheat toast	1 sl	51	2.4	10.8	0.7	55
Cottage cheese	1/2 cup (4 oz)	88	15.4	3.4	4.8	120
Water	1 cup	0	0.0	0.0	0.0	0
		326	33.0	26.6	17.3	394

* tr-trace (present, but too small to measure).

OR

You may eat for breakfast any of the lunches or dinners that have at least 28 gm of protein.

EASY NO-FLAB LUNCHES

20 "I CUT BACK ON CALORIES BY SKIPPING lunch." "I'm too busy to eat lunch." "I don't like paying restaurant prices for a low-calorie lunch, and we don't have facilities for brown-bagging at work, so I skip lunch." These are only a few of the reasons people give for skipping lunch.

Others eat too much. They can't resist all the tasty foods and desserts on the lunch menu, so they overeat. Or they're starved because they skipped breakfast, and they overeat. Or the homemaker may eat a good lunch, and then eat the kids' leftovers to prevent waste.

The biggest problem about lunch is developing a healthy attitude toward the noon meal. A nourishing lunch helps prevent fat storage and controls your appetite. Eating lunch keeps your blood sugar at the proper level. If you save 300 or 400 calories by skipping lunch, you will end up eating many times that amount in the next few days, because of the disruption in your blood-sugar level.

There's no such thing as a free lunch. One of the ways you pay for going overboard on a lunch—just because it's free—is to put on more fat. That spare tire around your waist may be the most expensive thing you own when you consider its cost in health problems and new wardrobe. You end up paying dearly for food that you think tasted doubly good because someone else picked up the check.

There are good lunches and bad lunches. Compare the nutrient level of a typical Easy No-Flab Lunch with a common lunch.

GUIDELINES FOR THE EASY NO-FLAB LUNCH

The Easy No-Flab Lunch Menu is even more flexible than the breakfast menu. The desired lunch contains about 333 FLAB Units, with nearly 1oz (at least 22 gm) of protein. Perfection would be 35 gm of protein, 35 gm of carbohydrate, and 13 gm of fat; however, lunch needn't be that exacting.

Lunch should complement breakfast and dinner, so that the entire day's menu provides an excellent nutritional balance. Each Easy No-Flab Lunch can be eaten with any of the Easy No-Flab Breakfasts or Dinners. That is, you can mix and match the various Breakfast, Lunch, and Dinner Menus as you like.

However, you may wish to choose your daily menus with regard to economy and convenience. As an example, if you have part of a melon, banana, or cup of yogurt for breakfast, you may wish to include the remainder in your lunch or dinner.

If you wonder "Why not eat all the yogurt at once, and switch the other foods for breakfast or dinner around to keep the calories at each meal the same?" you are missing the point of balancing the foods to keep the blood sugar at a reasonable level. Some foods contain too much of a single nutrient, and if large portions are to be eaten, they must be spread throughout the day by being blended into other meals.

TABLE 20-1–20-2 Lunch Comparisons

20-1

	Quantity	Prote (gm)	Carbo (gm)	Fat (gm)	Vit A
No-Flab Lunch					
Skim milk	3/4 cup	5.5	8.4	0.2	375
Whole wheat or Rye bread	1 sl	2.4	10.8	0.7	tr
Tossed salad	3/4 cup	0.7	2.7	0.1	1380
Beef & vegetable stew	1 cup	15.0	14.6	10.1	2303
Cottage cheese	2 oz	7.7	1.7	2.4	192
		31.3	38.2	13.5	4250
Typical Poor Lunch					
White bread	2 sl	4.0	23.0	1.4	0
Peanut butter	2 tbsp	8.9	5.5	15.8	0
Jelly	2 tbsp	0.0	24.5	0.0	0
Diet soda	1 bottle	0.0	tr*	0.0	0
		12.9	53.0	17.2	0

20-2

Lunch Comparisons

No-Flab Lunch	31.3	38.2	13.5	4,250
Poor Lunch	12.9	53.0	17.2	0

*tr-trace (present, but too small to measure).

Vit C	Vit B$_1$	Vit B$_2$	Vit B$_3$	Ca	Iron	Vit D	Cals
3.00	08	36	.16	228	.28	75	58
tr	09	06	.80	19	.60	0	55
26.00	03	04	.30	26	.60	0	13
16.00	14	16	4.50	28	2.80	0	209
.03	28	00	0.00	106	0.00	0	60
45.03	62	62	5.8	407	4.3	75	395
0	.18	.12	1.6	38	0.6	0	122
0	.04	.04	5.0	20	0.6	0	186
0	0.00	0.00	0.0	0	0.0	0	98
0	0.00	0.00	0.0	0	0.0	0	0
0	.22	.16	6.6	58	1.2	0	406
45	.62	.62	5.8	407	4.3	75	395
0	.22	.16	6.6	58	1.2	0	406

Easy No-Flab Lunch 1

Food	Quantity	FLABs	Prote (gm)	Carbo (gm)	Fat (gm)	Cals
Tossed Salad lettuce, carrot, green pepper, radish	3/4 cup	7	0.7	2.7	0.1	13
Beef and vegetable stew: 2 oz: beef, potato, peas, turnips, parsnips, celery, green pepper, onion, carrots	1 cup	179	15.0	14.6	10.1	209
Cottage cheese	2 oz	44	7.7	1.7	2.4	60
Whole wheat bread	1 sl	51	2.4	10.8	0.7	55
Skim milk	3/4 cup	46	5.5	8.4	0.2	58
Water	1 cup	0	0.0	0.0	0.0	0
		327	31.3	38.2	13.5	395

Sandwich shops and small coffee shops can provide nearly all of the lunches suggested, and essentially all can be obtained at restaurants or prepared at home. Brown-bag specials are lunches numbered 2, 4, 6, 11, 14, 20, and 21. Fast-food carry-out specials are numbers 7, 8, 10, and 16.

You might enjoy running through all twenty-one menus in consecutive order, but that's not necessary. The lunches can be eaten in any order you wish, or you can plan your own. *It is important for good nutrition, though, that you alternate between at least three different lunch menus.*

Easy No-Flab Lunch 2 (Brown-Bag Special)

Food	Quantity	FLABs	Prote (gm)	Carbo (gm)	Fat (gm)	Cals
Roast Beef Sandwich: 2 oz roast beef, 2 slices whole wheat or rye bread	1	184	21.8	21.6	6.8	231
Orange	1 med.	61	1.3	16.0	0.3	65
Skim milk	3/4 cup	46	5.5	8.4	0.2	58
Water	1 cup	0	0.0	0.0	0.0	0
		291	28.6	46.0	7.3	354

Easy No-Flab Lunch 3

Food	Quantity	FLABs	Prote (gm)	Carbo (gm)	Fat (gm)	Cals
Chicken noodle soup	1 cup	55	3.2	7.5	1.8	59
Ham, baked	3 oz	82	25.7	0.0	7.7	179
Pineapple Ring (water-pac)	1 small or 1/2 large	44	.2	10.7	.5	45
Whole wheat or Rye bread	1 sl	51	2.4	10.8	0.7	55
Skim milk	3/4 cup	46	5.5	8.4	0.2	58
Water	1 cup	0	0.0	0.0	0.0	0
		278	37.0	37.4	10.9	396

Easy No-Flab Lunch 4 (Brown-Bag Special)

Food	Quantity	FLABs	Prote (gm)	Carbo (gm)	Fat (gm)	Cals
Ham & cheese sandwich: 1 oz ham, 1 sl Swiss cheese, 2 slices whole wheat or Rye bread	1	186	17.4	21.9	7.8	221
Apple	1 med.	71	0.3	20.0	0.8	80
Skim milk	3/4 cup	46	5.5	8.4	0.2	58
Water	1 cup	0	0.0	0.0	0.0	0
		303	23.2	50.3	8.8	359
Men: Add another slice of Swiss Cheese		44	4.0	0.2	3.9	51
		347	27.2	50.5	12.7	410

You can design your own lunch around your favorite salads, soups, or sandwiches. Just be sure to include at least 250 FLAB Units and 22 gm of protein. As an upper limit, try not to go over 350 FLAB Units. The listing of FLAB Units in common foods is given in Appendix III.

If you find you are losing more than the weight recommended for you in Chapter 11, add more bread, milk, or fruit to your lunch to slow your weight-loss to the proper rate.

Remember: Breakfast like a king, but lunch like a prince.

Easy No-Flab Lunch 5

Food	Quantity	FLABs	Prote (gm)	Carbo (gm)	Fat (gm)	Cals
Breaded fish	3 oz	157	16.2	5.8	11.3	193
Peas, green	1/2 cup	52	4.1	9.4	0.2	54
Corn, canned	1/4 cup	27	1.1	8.2	0.4	35
Whole wheat bread	1 sl	51	2.4	10.8	0.7	55
Butter	1/2 tsp	18	tr*	tr	2.0	18
Skim milk	3/4 cup	46	5.5	8.4	0.2	58
Water	1 cup	0	0.0	0.0	0.0	0
		351	29.3	42.6	14.8	413

*tr- trace (present, but too small to measure).

Easy No-Flab Lunch 6 (Brown-Bag Special)

Food	Quantity	FLABs	Prote (gm)	Carbo (gm)	Fat (gm)	Cals
Yogurt	1/2 cup	103	4.6	21.0	1.1	113
Eggs, hard-boiled	2 lrg	134	13.0	1.0	11.6	164
Skim milk	1 cup	62	7.3	11.3	0.2	77
Water	1 cup	0	0.0	0.0	0.0	0
		299	24.9	33.3	12.9	354

Optional

Food	Quantity	FLABs	Prote (gm)	Carbo (gm)	Fat (gm)	Cals
Banana (Bing Cherries or Blueberries may be substituted for banana.)	1/2 med.	55	0.7	13.2	0.1	57
		354	25.6	46.5	13.0	411

Easy No-Flab Lunch 7 (Fast-Food Special)

Food	Quantity	FLABs	Prote (gm)	Carbo (gm)	Fat (gm)	Cals
Fried chicken Lunch (two types: one for men, one for women.)						
Women						
Fried chicken	2 oz	95	17.4	1.1	6.2	135
Coleslaw, with tbsp						
mayonnaise	1/2 cup	76	0.7	2.7	7.9	82
Corn,						
ear 4″ × 2″	1	70	3.3	21.0	1.0	91
Carrot, 5″	1	13	0.6	4.9	0.1	21
Skim milk	3/4 cup	46	5.5	8.4	0.2	58
Water	1 cup	0	0.0	0.0	0	0
		300	27.5	38.1	15.4	387
Men						
Fried chicken	3 oz	142	26.0	1.6	9.3	201
Coleslaw, with 1 tbsp						
mayonnaise	1/2 cup	76	0.7	2.7	7.9	82
Corn, ear,						
4″ × 2″	1	70	3.3	21.0	1.0	91
Skim milk	3/4 cup	46	5.5	8.4	0.2	58
Water	1 cup	0	0.0	0.0	0.0	0
		334	35.5	33.7	18.4	432

Easy No-Flab Lunch 8 (Fast-Food Special)

Food	Quantity	FLABs	Prote (gm)	Carbo (gm)	Fat (gm)	Cals
Salad, tossed	3/4 cup	7	0.7	2.7	0.1	13
Hamburger	3 oz	133	23.3	0.0	9.6	186
Hamburger roll	1	136	3.3	21.2	2.2	119
Skim milk	3/4 cup	46	5.5	8.4	0.2	58
Water	1 cup	0	0.0	0.0	0.0	0
		322	32.8	32.3	12.1	376
Men: Add another ounce of hamburger		44	7.7	0.0	3.2	61
		366	40.5	32.3	15.3	437

(an apple or pear can be substituted for tossed salad.)

Easy No-Flab Lunch 9

Food	Quantity	FLABs	Prote (gm)	Carbo (gm)	Fat (gm)	Cals
Chef's Salad: 1 oz turkey or chicken, 1/2 oz cheddar cheese, 1/2 egg, 1/2 tomato, 6 slices cucumber, 1/2 oz endive, 1/8 head lettuce, 1 tbsp salad dressing		281	39.5	17.1	14.9	342
Skim milk	3/4 cup	46	5.5	8.4	0.2	58
Water	1 cup	0	0.0	0.0	0.0	0
		327	45	25.5	15.1	400

Easy No-Flab Lunch 10 (Fast-Food Special)

Food	Quantity	FLABs (gm)	Prote (gm)	Carbo (gm)	Fat	Cals
Cheese pizza	5 oz (1/4 of 14")	328	18.0	42.5	12.5	354
Skim milk	3/4 cup	46	5.5	8.4	0.2	58
Water	1 cup	0	0.0	0.0	0.0	0
		374	23.5	50.9	12.7	412

Optional
Vegetable

Food	Quantity	FLABs (gm)	Prote (gm)	Carbo (gm)	Fat	Cals
juice	1/2 cup	25	1.1	5.2	0.1	26
		399	24.6	56.1	12.8	438

Easy No-Flab Lunch 11 (Brown-Bag Special)

Food	Quantity	FLABs	Prote (gm)	Carbo (gm)	Fat (gm)	Cals
Tuna fish salad sandwich	1	275	24.6	24.7	15.1	332
2 oz tuna,						
1/2 egg,						
1 tsp lemon juice,						
1 stalk celery,						
1 leaf lettuce,						
1 tbsp salad dressing,						
2 slices rye, Italian, or whole wheat bread						
Skim milk	3/4 cup	46	5.5	8.4	0.2	58
Water	1 cup	0	0.0	0.0	0.0	0
		321	30.1	33.1	15.3	390

Easy No-Flab Lunch 12

Food	Quantity	FLABs	Prote (gm)	Carbo (gm)	Fat (gm)	Cals
Grilled-cheese sandwich 2 slices whole wheat bread, 2 slices American cheese	1	268	16.8	24.8	17.8	318
Skim milk	3/4 cup	46	5.5	8.4	0.2	58
Water	1 cup	0	0.0	0.0	0.0	0
		314	22.3	33.2	18.0	376

Choice for Dieter
Either:
1/2 Apple
or
1/2 Pear or
1/2 cup vegetable
juice

Easy No-Flab Lunch 13

Food	Quantity	FLABs	Prote (gm)	Carbo (gm)	Fat (gm)	Cals
Cream of tomato soup	1 cup	173	6.5	22.5	7.0	173
Tuna	2 oz (1/3 cup)	74	16.4	0.0	4.6	112
Whole wheat bread	1 sl	51	2.4	10.8	0.7	55
Skim milk	3/4 cup	46	5.5	8.4	0.2	58
Water	1 cup	0	0.0	0.0	0.0	0
		344	30.8	41.7	12.5	398

Easy No-Flab Lunch 14 (Brown-Bag Special)

Food	Quantity	FLABs	Prote (gm)	Carbo (gm)	Fat (gm)	Cals
Chicken salad sandwich 1 oz chicken, 1 oz celery, 1 tbsp mayonnaise, and 2 slices whole wheat bread	1	262	33.5	23.0	13.0	329
Skim milk	3/4 cup	46	5.5	8.4	0.2	58
Water	1 cup	0	0.0	0.0	0.0	0
		308	39.0	31.4	13.2	387

Optional
Carrot or Celery sticks   1 or 2

Easy No-Flab Lunch 15

Food	Quantity	FLABs	Prote (gm)	Carbo (gm)	Fat (gm)	Cals
Tomato, stuffed with 5 oz cottage	1/2 med.	22	1.1	4.7	0.2	22
cheese	5/8 cup	108	19.0	4.1	6.0	150
Fruit salad	1/2 cup	96	1.5	24.8	0.5	110
Skim milk	1 cup	62	7.3	11.5	.2	77
Water	1 cup	0	0.0	0.0	0.0	0
		288	28.9	45.1	6.9	359

Dieter's
Choice
1/2 cup
Juice
or
1/2 med.
Fruit

Easy No-Flab Lunch 16 (Fast-Food Special)

Food	Quantity	FLABs	Prote (gm)	Carbo (gm)	Fat (gm)	Cals
Beef Taco: 1-1/2 oz beef, cheddar cheese, lettuce, tomato, corn tortilla	1 avg.	183	16.9	14.7	10.0	216
Apple	1 med.	71	0.3	20.0	0.8	80
Skim milk	1 cup	62	7.3	11.5	0.2	77
Water	1 cup	0	0.0	0.0	0.0	0
		316	24.5	46.2	11.0	373

OR

Food	Quantity	FLABs	Prote (gm)	Carbo (gm)	Fat (gm)	Cals
Beef taco (as above)	1 avg.	183	16.9	14.7	10.0	216
Yogurt	1/2 cup	103	4.6	21.0	1.1	113
Skim milk	1 cup	62	7.3	11.3	0.2	77
Water	1 cup	0	0.0	0.0	0.0	0
		348	28.8	47.0	11.3	406

Easy No-Flab Lunch 17

Food	Quantity	FLABs	Prote (gm)	Carbo (gm)	Fat (gm)	Cals
Chili con carne with beans	1/2 cup	154	9.4	15.3	7.7	167
Frankfurter, sliced (nitrate-free)	2 oz (1 avg.)	146	7.0	0.9	15.4	172
Skim milk	3/4 cup	46	5.5	8.4	0.2	58
Water	1 cup	0	0.0	0.0	0.0	0
		346	21.9	24.6	23.3	397

Easy No-Flab Lunch 18

Food	Quantity	FLABs	Prote (gm)	Carbo (gm)	Fat (gm)	Cals
Cheese Dream: 1 cover 1 sl of whole wheat bread with 1 sl of American cheese, warm until cheese softens, spread 2 oz (1/4 cup) cottage cheese or a cheese spread on top. Sprinkle with chopped walnuts if desired.		178	16.1	14.2	11.3	219
Banana or Pear	1 med.	111	1.3	26.4	0.2	101
Water	1 cup	0	0.0	0.0	0.0	0
Skim milk	3/4 cup	46	5.5	8.4	0.2	58
		335	22.9	49	11.7	378

Easy No-Flab Lunch 19

Food	Quantity	FLABs	Prote (gm)	Carbo (gm)	Fat (gm)	Cals
Cream of tomato soup	1 cup	173	6.5	22.5	7.0	173
Turkey slices	2 oz	79	18.6	0.0	4.6	120
Butter	1/2 tsp	18	tr*	tr	2.0	18
Whole wheat bread	1 sl	51	2.4	10.8	0.7	55
Skim milk	3/4 cup	46	5.5	8.4	0.2	58
Water	1 cup	0	0.0	0.0	0.0	0
		367	33	41.7	14.5	424

*tr-trace (present, but too small to measure).

Easy No-Flab Lunch 20 (Brown-Bag Special)

Food	Quantity	FLABs	Prote (gm)	Carbo (gm)	Fat (gm)	Cals
Peanut Butter and cheese, open-face: spread 2 tbsp peanut butter on 1 sl of whole wheat bread, cover with 1 sl American cheese	1	325	17.3	17.9	24.7	345
Skim milk	3/4 cup	46	5.5	8.4	0.2	58
Water	1 cup	0	0.0	0.0	0.0	0
		371	22.8	26.3	24.9	403

Optional
1/2 cup
vegetable
juice
or
2 to 3 car-
rot sticks

Easy No-Flab Lunch 21 (Brown-Bag Special)

Food	Quantity	FLABs	Prote (gm)	Carbo (gm)	Fat (gm)	Cals
Sardines in mustard	1/2 can	92	11.0	0.0	8.0	115
Apple	1/2 med.	71	0.3	20.0	0.8	80
Whole wheat bread	2 sl	102	4.8	21.6	1.4	110
Skim milk	1 cup	62	7.3	11.3	7.3	77
Water	1 cup	0	0.0	0.0	0.0	0
		327	23.4	52.9	17.5	382

Easy No-Flab Lunch 22

Any No-Flab breakfasts or dinner menus. Don't forget the quick 5-minute blender "milkshake" meals.

EASY NO-FLAB DINNERS

21 STUDIES HAVE SHOWN THAT FOOD EAT-
en after our active part of the day is mostly converted to fat. Food with the same number of calories eaten before the end of our day's major activities is
burned with no weight-gain.

The Easy No-Flab Diet is designed to distribute food
evenly throughout your day's activities. This will help
keep your blood-sugar level constant and so keep you full
of energy and free of hunger.

The Easy No-Flab Diet is different from most diets,
which give you only 150 to 200 calories for breakfast or
lunch, but then suggest a dinner of 600 to 700 calories.

You will lose more fat faster, while eating more food,
on the Easy No-Flab Diet than you will on a lower calorie
diet that encourages eating meals that are unbalanced in
food quantity and nutrients.

I have urged you to breakfast like a king, and lunch like
a prince. At your evening meal it's time to dine like a
pauper. But that's okay. You won't be so hungry anyway.

We tend to eat too much at dinner. This excess over-
whelms our body's ability to handle or transport the food
components. Our blood becomes saturated with fatty

172

chemicals that can be deposited as fat in fat cells or in fat deposits in our arteries. Those deposits can cause heart disease and other serious health problems. Our ability to work and exercise decreases, and a heart attack can be triggered.

In short, little can be said in benefit of gorging at dinner. It's better for you to eat dinners about the size of your breakfast and lunches.

GUIDELINES FOR DINNER

Ideally, dinner should contain about 333 FLAB Units, with 35 gm of protein. A more practical goal would be dinners in the 275- to 350-FLAB Unit range, with at least 28 gm of protein, and about 30 to 40 gm of carbohydrates.

The following twenty-one menus are only suggestions of the countless variations you can design keeping the Easy No-Flab Diet Dinner Guidelines in mind.

You might even enjoy trying all twenty-one menus in consecutive order.

Try as many variations as you like.

Use at least five different Easy No-Flab Dinner menu variations on a rotating basis.

Keep your meals interesting and be sure that you get all types of food. Fast-Food specials are numbered 16 and 18.

Because some important nutrients may not have been identified yet, you would eat a variety of foods to be sure you're not missing something that's good for you.

Easy No-Flab Dinner 1

Food	Quantity	FLABs	Prote (gm)	Carbo (gm)	Fat (gm)	Cals
Fillet of flounder	4 oz (uncooked)	49	20.0	0.0	1.0	85
Mashed potato	1/2 cup	63	2.1	12.3	4.3	74
Asparagus spears with lemon slices	4	11	1.3	2.2	0.1	12
Butter	1 tsp	36	0.0	0.0	4.1	36
Tossed salad: lettuce, carrot, green pepper, radish	3/4 cup	7	0.7	2.7	0.1	13
Salad dressing (French or Thousand Island)	3/4 tbsp	50	0.1	2.1	3.1	50
Whole wheat bread or other whole grain	1 sl	51	2.4	10.8	0.7	55
Skim milk	3/4 cup	46	5.5	8.4	0.2	58
Water	1 cup	0	0.0	0.0	0.0	0
		313	32.1	38.5	13.6	383

Men: add another teaspoon of butter for mashed potato or bread, if you want.

Easy No-Flab Dinner 2

Food	Quantity	FLABs	Prote (gm)	Carbo (gm)	Fat (gm)	Cals
Rib lamb chop, broiled	3 oz	196	21.4	0.0	17.0	242
Rice	1/3 cup	71	1.4	16.5	0.1	75
Tossed salad: lettuce, carrot, green pepper, radish	3/4 cup	7	0.7	2.7	0.1	13
Skim milk	3/4 cup	46	5.5	8.4	0.2	58
Water	1 cup	0	0.0	0.0	0.0	0
		320	29.0	27.6	17.4	388

Men: add a sl of whole wheat or other whole grain bread, if you like.

Easy No-Flab Dinner 3

Food	Quantity	FLABs	Prote (gm)	Carbo (gm)	Fat (gm)	Cals
Roast turkey	4 oz (3 med. sl)	157	37.2	0.0	9.2	240
Sweet potato, baked	1/2 med.	68	1.2	17.9	0.3	78
Asparagus, cooked	4 spears	11	1.3	2.2	0.1	12
Lettuce leaves	2 lrg	4	0.7	1.8	0.2	9
Tomato	3 sl	22	1.1	4.7	0.2	22
Skim milk	3/4 cup	46	5.5	8.4	0.2	58
Water	1 cup	0	0.0	0.0	0.0	0
		308	47	35	10.2	419

Men: add a half sl of whole wheat or rye bread, if you want.

Easy No-Flab Dinner 4

Food	Quantity	FLABs	Prote (gm)	Carbo (gm)	Fat (gm)	Cals
Calves' liver, broiled	3 oz	144	22.5	4.5	9.0	195
Onions, sliced	1/3 cup	16	0.9	4.5	0.1	84
Sweet potato, baked	1/2 med.	68	1.2	17.9	0.3	78
Skim milk	3/4 cup	46	5.5	8.4	0.2	58
Water	1 cup	0	0.0	0.0	0.0	0
		274	30.1	35.3	9.6	415

Men: add a half slice of whole wheat bread, if you like.

Easy No-Flab Dinner 5

Food	Quantity	FLABs	Prote (gm)	Carbo (gm)	Fat (gm)	Cals
Sirloin strip steak	3 oz (cooked)	130	22.0	0.0	9.5	180
Baked potato (or Macaroni salad)	1/2 lrg	62	1.9	14.9	0.1	70
Beets with greens	1/2 cup	30	0.8	7.3	0.1	31
Tossed salad: lettuce, carrot, green pepper, radish	3/4 cup	7	0.7	2.7	0.1	31
French dressing	1 tbsp	65	0.1	2.8	6.2	66
Skim milk	3/4 cup	46	5.5	8.4	0.2	58
Water	1 cup	0	0.0	0.0	0.0	0
		340	31	36.1	16.2	418

Men: add a half slice of whole wheat or rye bread, if you like.

Easy No-Flab Dinner 6

Food	Quantity	FLABs	Prote (gm)	Carbo (gm)	Fat (gm)	Cals
Roasted chicken	4 oz cooked meat (9 oz uncooked with skin and bones)	138	35.2	0.0	7.5	218
Baked potato or potato salad	1/2 lrg	62	1.9	14.9	0.1	70
Butter	1 tsp	36	0.0	0.0	4.1	36
Tossed salad: lettuce, carrot, green pepper, radish	3/4 cup	7	0.7	2.7	0.1	13
Green beans	1/2 cup	15	1.0	3.4	0.1	16
Skim milk	3/4 cup	46	5.5	8.4	0.2	58
Water	1 cup	0	0.0	0.0	0.0	0
		304	44.3	29.4	12.1	411

Men: add a half
slice of whole wheat or other whole grain bread.

Easy No-Flab Dinner 7

Food	Quantity	FLABs	Prote (gm)	Carbo (gm)	Fat (gm)	Cals
Red snapper, broiled	5 oz cooked (7 oz uncooked)	100	41.6	0.0	1.9	195
Butter	1 tsp	36	0.0	0.0	4.1	36
Rice	1/2 cup	106	2.1	24.8	0.1	112
Beets, diced	1/2 cup	30	0.8	7.3	0.1	31
Skim milk	3/4 cup	46	5.5	8.4	0.2	58
Water	1 cup	0	0.0	0.0	0.0	0
		318	50.0	40.5	6.4	431

Alternative for beets
Summer squash
Soybean sprouts

Easy No-Flab Dinner 8

Food	Quantity	FLABs	Prote (gm)	Carbo (gm)	Fat (gm)	Cals
Beef, top round	3 oz cooked (4 oz uncooked)	169	24.6	0.0	13.3	225
Noodles (egg)	1/2 cup	95	3.3	18.6	1.2	100
Carrots, cooked	1/2 cup	18	0.7	5.1	0.1	22
Green pepper	1/4 lrg	5	0.3	1.2	0.5	5
Skim milk	3/4 cup	46	5.5	8.4	0.2	58
Water	1 cup	0	0.0	0.0	0.0	0
		333	34.4	33.3	15.3	410

Men: May add a half slice of whole wheat bread.

Easy No-Flab Dinner 9

Food	Quantity	FLABs	Prote (gm)	Carbo (gm)	Fat (gm)	Cals
Baked ham	3 oz	121	25.7	0.0	7.7	179
Pineapple ring	1 lrg	90	0.4	23.7	0.1	90
Peas, black-eye	1/3 cup	82	6.7	14.9	0.7	89
Skim milk	3/4 cup	46	5.5	8.4	0.2	58
Water	1 cup	0	0.0	0.0	0.0	0
		339	38.3	47	8.7	416

Easy No-Flab Dinner 10

Food	Quantity	FLABs	Prote (gm)	Carbo (gm)	Fat (gm)	Cals
T-bone steak	3 1/2 oz	146	29.0	0.0	9.8	212
Potatoes, boiled	2 small	72	2.3	17.7	0.1	81
Carrots, cooked or raw	1/2 cup	18	0.7	5.1	0.1	22
Lettuce leaves	2 lrg	4	0.7	1.8	0.2	9
Tomato	1 sl	7	0.4	1.6	0.1	7
Whole wheat bread	1/2 sl	26	1.2	5.4	0.4	28
Skim milk	3/4 cup	46	5.5	8.4	0.2	58
Water	1 cup	0	0.0	0.0	0.0	0
		319	39.8	40	10.9	417

Men: may add a tsp of butter.

Easy No-Flab Dinner 11

Food	Quantity	FLABs	Prote (gm)	Carbo (gm)	Fat (gm)	Cals
Hamburger, broiled	3 oz cooked	133	23.3	0.0	9.6	186
Potato, baked (or potato salad)	1/2 lrg	62	1.9	14.9	0.1	70
Lima beans	1/2 cup	89	6.5	16.8	0.4	94
Tomato	1 small	7	0.4	1.6	0.1	7
Skim milk	3/4 cup	46	5.5	8.4	0.2	58
Water	1 cup	0	0.0	0.0	0.0	0
		337	37.6	41.7	10.4	415

Men: may add a half sl of whole wheat or rye bread.

Easy No-Flab Dinner 12

Food	Quantity	FLABs	Prote (gm)	Carbo (gm)	Fat (gm)	Cals
Baked veal loin chop	3 1/2 oz cooked (6 oz raw with bone)	135	35.8	0.0	7.0	217
Rice, cooked	1/2 cup	106	2.1	24.8	0.1	112
Stewed tomatoes	1/2 cup	22	1.1	4.7	0.2	22
Okra (or tossed salad as in earlier menus) as in earlier menus)	1/2 cup	10	0.9	2.6	0.1	12
Skim milk	3/4 cup	46	5.5	8.4	0.2	58
Water	1 cup	0	0.0	0.0	0.0	0
		319	45.4	40.5	7.6	421

Men: may add a half sl of whole wheat or rye bread.

Easy No-Flab Dinner 13

Food	Quantity	FLABs	Prote (gm)	Carbo (gm)	Fat (gm)	Cals
Roast beef, top round	3 oz	124	25.5	0.0	8.1	182
Baked potato	1 lrg	123	3.7	29.9	0.1	132
Butter	1 tsp	36	0.0	0.0	4.1	36
Zucchini	1/2 cup	12	1.0	2.5	0.1	12
Skim milk	3/4 cup	46	5.5	8.4	0.2	58
Water	1 cup	0	0.0	0.0	0.0	0
		341	35.7	40.8	12.6	420

Men: may add a half sl of whole wheat bread.

Easy No-Flab Dinner 14

Food	Quantity	FLABs	Prote (gm)	Carbo (gm)	Fat (gm)	Cals
Trout, Bluefish or Perch, baked Fillet	4 1/2 oz cooked (6 oz raw)	141	36.8	0.0	7.5	225
Potato, mashed	1/2 cup	63	2.0	12.7	0.7	74
Broccoli with lemon juice	1/2 cup (1 stalk)	23	2.4	3.5	0.2	26
Beets, cooked, sliced	1/2 cup	30	0.8	7.3	0.1	31
Skim milk	3/4 cup	46	5.5	8.4	0.2	58
Water	1 cup	0	0.0	0.0	0.0	0
		303	47.5	31.9	8.7	414

Men: may add a half sl of whole wheat or rye bread.

Easy No-Flab Dinner 15

Food	Quantity	FLABs	Prote (gm)	Carbo (gm)	Fat (gm)	Cals
Bottom round	3 oz	134	30.4	0.0	8.1	203
Potatoes, boiled	2 small	72	2.3	17.7	0.1	81
Broccoli with butter	1 stalk	23	2.4	3.5	0.2	26
	1 tsp	36	0.0	4.1	0.0	36
Celery	8"	2	0.5	2.2	0.1	10
Carrots, raw, stick	5"	13	0.6	4.9	0.1	21
Skim milk	3/4 cup	46	5.5	8.4	0.2	58
Water	1 cup	0	0.0	0.0	0.0	0
		326	41.7	40.8	8.8	435

Easy No-Flab Dinner 16 (Fast-Food Special)

Food	Quantity	FLABs	Prote (gm)	Carbo (gm)	Fat (gm)	Cals
Breaded fish or Fish sticks with lemon wedge	4 oz	209	21.5	7.7	15.0	257
Corn on the cob (5" × 1 3/4")	1	87	4.1	26.3	1.3	114
Skim milk	3/4 cup	46	5.5	8.4	0.2	58
Water	1 cup	0	0.0	0.0	0.0	0
		342	31.1	42.4	16.5	429

Easy No-Flab Dinner 17

Food	Quantity	FLABs	Prote (gm)	Carbo (gm)	Fat (gm)	Cals
Meat loaf	3 1/2 oz	228	18.4	14.8	14.5	268
Peas, green	1/2 cup	52	4.1	9.4	0.2	54
Skim milk	3/4 cup	45	5.5	8.4	0.2	58
Water	1 cup	0	0.0	0.0	0.0	0
		325	28.0	32.6	14.9	380
Men: may add mashed potato	1/4 cup	32	1.0	6.4	0.4	37
and butter	1 tsp	36	0.0	0.0	4.1	36
		393	29	39	19.4	453

Easy No-Flab Dinner 18 (Fast-Food Special)

Food	Quantity	FLABs	Prote (gm)	Carbo (gm)	Fat (gm)	Cals
Fried chicken	5 oz (leg, thigh)	142	26.0	1.6	9.3	201
Coleslaw with mayonnaise	1/2 cup	76	0.7	2.7	7.9	82
Corn, ear (5" × 1 3/4")	1	87	4.1	26.3	1.3	114
Skim milk	3/4 cup	46	5.5	8.4	0.2	58
Water	1 cup	0	0.0	0.0	0.0	0
		351	36.3	39	18.7	455

Easy No-Flab Dinner 19

Food	Quantity	FLABs	Prote (gm)	Carbo (gm)	Fat (gm)	Cals
Baked rib veal chop	4 oz	157	38.2	0.0	9.0	245
Corn	1/2 cup	54	2.2	16.4	0.7	70
Greens, cooked (mustard greens, spinach greens, turnip greens	1/2 cup	15	1.9	2.9	0.2	17
Onion	1/4 cup	12	0.7	3.4	0.1	15
Whole wheat bread	1 sl	51	2.4	10.8	0.7	55
Skim milk	3/4 cup	46	5.5	8.4	0.2	58
Water	1 cup	0	0.0	0.0	0.0	0
		335	50.9	41.9	10.9	460

Easy No-Flab Dinner 20

Food	Quantity	FLABs	Prote (gm)	Carbo (gm)	Fat (gm)	Cals
Spaghetti, Meatballs, Romano cheese, and tomato sauce	1/2 cup	154	9.3	19.4	5.9	166
Extra Meatballs	1 oz	60	10.7	2.3	3.1	82
Tossed salad (as earlier)	3/4 cup	7	0.7	2.7	0.1	13
Italian bread	1 sl	51	2.4	10.8	0.7	55
Skim milk	3/4 cup	46	5.5	8.4	0.2	58
Water	1 cup	0	0.0	0.0	0.0	0
		318	28.6	43.6	10	374

Men: may add a tsp of butter.

Easy No-Flab Dinner 21

Food	Quantity	FLABs	Prote (gm)	Carbo (gm)	Fat (gm)	Cals
Mashed potato	1/2 cup	64	2.0	12.8	0.8	64
Tossed salad (as earlier)	3/4 cup	7	0.7	2.7	0.1	13
Skim milk	3/4 cup	46	5.5	8.4	0.2	58
Water	1 cup	0	0.0	0.0	0.0	0
Carrot Coins Beef Loaf	1 serving	239	20.4	15.6	15.3	282
		356	28.6	39.5	16.4	417

RECIPE

Carrot Coins Beef Loaf*
2 pounds ground beef (80 percent lean)
5 long carrots
1 can (16 oz) tomatoes
1 3/4 tsp salt
1 1/8 tsp leaf oregano
1/4 tsp pepper
1/2 cup crushed crackers
2 med. onions, cut in 1/4" slices
1 egg
1 small green pepper, cut in thin strips
1 cup sliced celery
1/2 cup water
1 tbsp cornstarch

Cook carrots (whole) in boiling salted water in large covered frying pan 15 minutes; drain. Drain tomatoes, reserving juice; cut tomatoes into large pieces. Stir 3/4 cup of reserved tomato juice, 1 1/2 tsp salt, 1 tsp oregano and pepper into cracker crumbs in large bowl. Chop enough onion slices to make 1/4 cup. Add ground beef, chopped onion and egg to cracker-crumb mixture; mix lightly but thoroughly. Place 1/3 of mixture in 9" × 5" loaf pan, pressing into layer in bottom of pan. Place 2 carrots lengthwise in pan and press into meat mixture. Top with layer of second 1/3 of meat mixture. Place 1 carrot down the center and press into meat. Add remaining meat mixture to form layer and press last 2 carrots into top, covering them with meat. Bake in a moderate oven (350°F.) for 1 hour 15 minutes or until done.

For vegetable sauce, add remaining onion slices, green pepper, celery, 1/4 tsp salt and 1/8 tsp oregano to boiling water in saucepan. Cover tightly and cook 15 minutes or until vegetables are almost tender. Combine cornstarch with remaining reserved tomato juice and pieces of tomatoes. Gradually combine with vegetables and cook 3 to 5 minutes,

*Recipe courtesy of National Livestock and Meat Board

stirring until thickened. Slice meat loaf in 10 equal slices and serve with vegetable sauce. 10 servings of 1 slice each.

OR

Any of the Easy No-Flab Breakfasts or Lunches having more than 28 gm of protein can be enjoyed for dinner.

NO-FLAB SNACKS

SNACKS ARE A KEY PART OF THE EASY No-Flab Diet. Snacks at midmorning and midafternoon will prevent the blood-sugar level from plummeting. It's that plunge that causes the hunger pangs that ruin most attempts at dieting.

If you snack, you can eat smaller meals. Smaller meals will keep your blood sugar at reasonable levels and thus prevent fat storage. Consistent smaller meals will reset your appestat properly over a period of time. Some people even think the evenness of several frequent small meals allows their stomach to "shrink back to normal." They may be right.

Snacks are especially critical during the first 7 to 10 days of the diet, but after that they can be slowly reduced if your body tells you that you feel too full, or if it's inconvenient for you to snack because of work or travel schedules.

Use snacks to "fine tune" your rate of fat-loss. If you are losing too fast after 2 or 3 weeks, increase the amount in your snacks. If you are not meeting your charted goals, skip the snack you feel you can best do without.

Hypoglycemics and those with a strong sweet tooth will usually do best keeping at least one snack throughout the duration of their diet.

TWO DAYTIME SNACKS

At the midmorning and midafternoon snacks, drink at least 1 8-oz glass of water (preferably filtered or bottled water). Men should eat a slice of cheese or a hard-boiled egg. Recent studies have shown that eating eggs does *not* effect the blood cholesterol levels of most healthy individuals receiving proper nutrition and moderate exercise, such as in the Easy No-Flab Diet.* Individuals with elevated blood cholesterol levels usually will achieve normalization on this diet. However, those with elevated cholesterol or triglycerides should have them measured during the diet. Women should eat a half slice of cheese or half of a hard-boiled egg with their glass of water.

The water is vitally needed for the life processes and is also needed to give the proper consistency to the roughage (fiber) in the bowel to prevent constipation. Diets cut back on the food eaten and the bulk, but few people realize that they have also cut back on their water because water is the largest component of most foods. If you don't like drinking water, try mixing in a teaspoon of lemon or lime juice. Even a teaspoon of lemonade mixed in the glass of water would be okay. You'll soon prefer the "weak" juice over full-strength juices or lemonade, and they're better for you.

---

*(Flynn et al., *The American Journal of Clinical Nutrition*, 1051–1057, May 1979;
Slater et al., *Nutrition Reports International*, 1976;
Kummerow et al., *The American Journal of Clinical Nutrition*, 1977.

THE NIGHTTIME SNACK

In the evening, after you've exercised or as you wind down preparing for bed, you should have a cup of unsalted, unbuttered popcorn. Pop the corn in butter or oil, but don't use any butter or oil on the kernels for flavoring. You can pop a lot of corn at one time and store it for several days in plastic bags, or you can buy pre-popped, unsalted, unbuttered corn.

Popcorn is not fully digestible and adds needed bulk to your No-Flab Diet. This helps maintain the "full" sensation from the intestines that helps your appestat determine that you have eaten sufficiently, and turns off your hunger.

If you don't want to mess with the popcorn, unsweetened "puffed" cereal or 4 stalks of celery can be substituted. After the first 7 to 10 days, your blood sugar will be well under control and then you can vary your snacks or cut back, if you wish.

SNACK VARIATIONS

Regardless of which snacks you choose, or even if you omit them later, you will still need to drink the water at midmorning, midafternoon and at bedtime. You may substitute any of the following for any snack after the first 7 to 10 days of the diet.

Nuts and Seeds
  2 tsp of sunflower or pumpkin seeds
  10 lrg peanuts
  7 almonds
Fruits
  6 fresh grapes
  1/4 med. apple
  1/2 orange
  1/4 fresh pear

1/2 tangerine
5 fresh strawberries
1/4 cup unsweetened cubed pineapple
1/2 fresh peach
Vegetables (no limit)
Cauliflowerets
Celery sticks
Cherry tomatoes
Zucchini sticks
Green pepper strips
Carrot sticks
Radishes
Cabbage pieces (bite-size)
Lettuce
Parsley
Watercress
Bean sprouts
Alfalfa sprouts
Cucumber
Asparagus spears
Endive
Beverages (snacks, but not substitutes for the water)
1 cup unsweetened, weak iced or hot tea spiced with ginger root or cinnamon stick
1/2 cup tomato juice blended with 1/2 cup sliced cucumber, 1/8 crushed dried mint, and dash of Tabasco.

Remember that for the first 7 to 10 days, three snacks a day are required. After that initial period snacks are optional. You can even use them for rewards as you lose each pound. Many of these snacks make excellent party snacks as well as diet snacks. There is never a need to go hungry. The idea is to lose flab—not torture yourself. You will be amazed at how tasty snacks can be without having to resort to junk food. Good nutrition can be tasty and dieting can be painless. Enjoy!

NO-FLAB DIET SHAKES—
WHEN YOU DON'T
HAVE TIME TO EAT

23 YOU CAN REPLACE OCCASIONAL BREAK-
fasts and lunches on the Easy No-Flab Diet Program with either a delicious milkshake or juice-
shake that tastes like a sherbert. These Diet Shakes are
made by adding protein powder and optional flavors to
milk or fruit juice. The protein Diet Shakes should not be
confused with the liquid predigested-protein diet, which
must be closely supervised by specially trained physicians.

It is important to eat two well-balanced No-Flab meals
any day you have one Diet Shake Meal. The two No-Flab
meals are necessary to provide the nutrients not in the
protein powder, milk, or orange juice.

You can make your own protein powder by mixing
equal parts of powdered eggs and dried milk, but the com-
mercial protein powders, made from soybean protein,
mix more easily with milk or juice and are more palat-
able.

192

DIET SHAKES—PRO AND CON

The Easy No-Flab Diet Program is the best reducing-diet program I know of for most people. However, no diet will be perfect for everyone. Some people can't always prepare their breakfast or lunch for one reason or another. Others will not eat good food three meals a day. And some will insist on losing weight faster than they should. It's far better that those people who are tempted to skip a meal have a Diet Shake, rather than no food at all.

Diet Shakes have several good features:

1. They are safe.
2. They provide less opportunity to cheat on food proportions.
3. They can be prepared rapidly.
4. They provide adequate protein.
5. There are many delicious variations.
6. They cost less than coffee and donuts, and
7. Each Diet Shake is a complete meal.

Diet Shakes do have disadvantages:

1. Hunger will be slightly greater for the first week or so because of the uneven balance of food proportions you will be eating at breakfast, lunch, and dinner, and
2. Good eating habits will be disrupted.

WHERE TO GET PROTEIN POWDER AND HOW TO USE IT

Protein powder is versatile because it can be mixed with liquids or added to solids, it's easily stored without refrigeration, and requires no cooking.

Numerous brands of protein powders are available in health food stores and many drug stores. Or you can prepare your own. Some of the brands will have slightly better quality of protein mixtures than others, or have the superior quality of added nutrients. That is more critical when you consistently drink Diet Shakes twice a day for many weeks at a time. Since I am suggesting only occasional use of the Diet Shakes, always complemented by two daily No-Flab meals, you will find that all brands will be adequate, but one brand may appeal to you over another because of mixing characteristics or flavor.

Small amounts of fructose (fruit sugar) or honey can be added to the protein powder as a sweetener without affecting your insulin secretion seriously, provided that you are not diabetic or hypoglycemic. Diabetics should not use honey, nor should some hypoglycemics. Some diabetics may find that fructose is useful as a low-insulin-secreting carbohydrate, **if used sparingly.** However, diabetics and hypoglycemics should exercise caution while testing their individual response to fructose.

Some protein powders come premixed with fructose, or fructose can be purchased at health food stoes and some drug stores.

Most protein-powder diet plans recommend mixing the protein powder with skim milk because of the lower calorie content of skim milk, but I prefer to use low-fat (2 percent butterfat) or whole milk, or better yet, skim milk plus lecithin* to increase the calorie level to prevent too rapid weight-loss, which would remove lean tissue as well as flab.

---

*Lecithin is a healthful food supplement important in fat metabolism. It is available from health food stores. It is a very rich source of calories, so only add a teaspoon per Diet Shake.

YOU NOTICE I DID NOT SAY LIQUID PRE-DIGESTED PROTEIN

The liquid predigested protein diet is exclusively a protein diet that is very low in calories. It has its advantages for those who can't lose weight by other means. **However, the liquid predigested diet should only be used under the close supervision of a specially trained physician. A low-calorie diet of anything—liquid protein, steak, eggs, carrots, or candy bars—can be fatal because of the danger of malnutrition.**

Liquid predigested protein is not a high-quality food for nutritional purposes, but the product has important uses as a protein supplement for patients unable to eat protein foods normally. It is only the use of liquid predigested protein alone—without other foods for dieting purposes without the proper medical supervision—to which I object.

The Diet Shakes that replace breakfast or lunch have 161 FLAB Units, 218 calories, 35.7 gm of protein, 11.3 gm of carbohydrates, and 4.9 gm of fat, when 1 oz of protein powder is mixed with 1 cup of low-fat (2 percent butterfat) milk.

If you find it advantageous to drink breakfast or lunch, add the cheese and milk snack if weight-loss is too rapid, or if hunger is a problem. On any day that you use a Diet Shake, you should make sure that you get all six glasses of water that are part of the Easy No-Flab Diet.

You can add variety to the Diet Shakes by concocting different milkshake or fruitshake recipes. Here are just a few suggestions developed at Weight Loss International® and reprinted with their permission. I was Nutritional Advisor and Director of Research and Development for Weight Loss International before developing the Easy No-Flab Diet and observed how these Diet Shakes helped hundreds of thousands of people take off unwanted pounds.

Banana Shake
8 oz of milk
2 tbsp protein powder
1 tsp banana extract
1/2 tsp honey or fructose
a few ice cubes

Fruit Juicy Shake
6 oz unsweetened or dietetic juice such as orange, cranberry, cran-apple, grapefruit
2 tbsp protein powder
1/2 tsp honey or fructose
a few ice cubes

Triple Fruit Cooler
2 oz milk
2 tbsp protein powder
6 oz orange juice
1/2 tsp banana or pineapple extract
4 fresh or frozen strawberries
1/2 tsp honey or fructose
2–4 ice cubes

Cherry Flip
8 oz milk
2 tbsp protein powder
1 tsp rum or brandy extract
1 tsp cherry extract
1/2 tsp honey or fructose
2–4 ice cubes
Sprinkle with nutmeg

Shirley Temple
4 oz milk
2 tbsp protein powder
4 oz orange juice
1 tbsp lemon juice
1 tsp cherry extract
1/2 tsp honey or fructose
2–4 ice cubes

Nevada Cocktail
2 tbsp protein powder
6 oz grapefruit juice
1 tbsp lemon juice
1 tsp rum extract
1/2 tsp honey or fructose
2–4 ice cubes

Strawberry Shake
8 oz milk
2 tbsp protein powder
1 tsp strawberry extract or fresh or frozen strawberries
1/2 tsp fructose or honey
2–4 ice cubes

Florida Cooler
8 oz milk
2 tbsp protein powder
1/2 tsp each pineapple & banana extract
1/2 tsp honey or fructose
2–4 ice cubes
Sprinkle with nutmeg

Peach Shake
8 oz milk
2 tbsp protein powder
1 fresh peach
1/2 tsp honey or fructose
2–4 cubes

Fruit Salute
2 tbsp protein powder
4 oz water
4 oz orange juice
1 tbsp lemon juice
1 tsp pineapple extract
1 tsp rum extract
1/2 tsp honey or fructose
2–4 ice cubes

Cape Codler
2 tbsp protein powder
5 oz cranberry juice
1 oz lime juice
1 tsp rum extract
1/2 tsp honey or fructose
2–4 ice cubes

La Jolla
4 oz milk
2 tbsp protein powder
1 tbsp lemon juice
2 oz orange juice
1/2 tsp banana extract
1/2 tsp honey or fructose
2–4 ice cubes

Mocha Shake
8 oz milk
2 tbsp protein powder
1/2 tsp decaffeinated instant coffee
1/2 tsp chocolate extract
1/2 tsp honey or fructose
a few ice cubes

Creamsickle Shake
8 oz milk
2 tbsp protein powder
1/2 tsp orange extract
1/2 tsp vanilla extract
1/2 tsp honey or fructose
a few ice cubes

Black Forest Shake
8 oz milk
2 tbsp protein powder
1/2 tsp chocolate extract
1/2 tsp black walnut extract
1/2 tsp honey or fructose
a few ice cubes

Piña Colada Shake

8 oz milk
2 tbsp protein powder
1/2–1 tsp coconut extract
1/2 tsp rum extract
1/2 tsp honey or fructose
3–4 ice cubes

Vanilla Butter & Nut

8 oz milk
2 tbsp protein powder
1 tsp vanilla
Butter & nut extract
Dash of cinnamon
1/2 tsp honey or fructose
Serve hot or cold

Coffee Mint

8 oz milk
2 tbsp protein powder
2 tsp decaffeinated instant coffee
1/2 tsp mint extract
1/2 tsp honey or fructose
2–4 ice cubes

Brandy Alexander

8 oz milk
2 tbsp protein powder
1 tsp brandy extract
1/2 tsp honey or fructose
2–4 ice cubes

Brandy Alexander's Sister

8 oz milk
2 tbsp protein powder
1 tsp brandy extract
1/2 tsp mint extract
1/2 tsp honey or fructose
2–4 ice cubes

DIET SHAKES FOR MAINTENANCE

Diet Shakes can be used to help maintain your desired weight. If you notice your weight beginning to creep up, you can reverse the process quickly before it gets out of hand by using a Diet Shake in place of a meal for a day or two. There is no need to gear up for a diet. Just reduce calories for a day or two by using the Diet Shakes. Chapter 27 offers advice on maintaining ideal weight.

NO-FLAB VITAMINS AND FOOD SUPPLEMENTS

(24) IT MAKES GOOD SENSE TO TAKE A QUAL-
ity vitamin and mineral supplement regularly.
In general it's an economical investment in
your health.

During periods of dieting, a vitamin and mineral supplement is a necessity. Not only is your food quantity,
and thus your nutrient intake, restricted, there are additional physical and mental stresses that rob your body of
the nutrients it needs. Furthermore, most reducing diets
are deficient in iron, calcium, and the B-Complex vitamins.

TOO FEW VITAMINS WILL SLOW YOUR FAT-LOSS

A vitamin or mineral deficiency will slow the conversion of body fat to energy; so, if you are undernourished,
you will not lose fat so fast as you would if you were well
nourished. Also, if you are undernourished, your body
will crave more food in a subconscious effort to get more
nutrients.

TOO MANY VITAMINS WON'T SPEED YOUR FAT-LOSS

This is not to say that even more vitamins and minerals will help you lose weight still faster. Extra vitamins and minerals above the official recommended daily allowances for the average person may benefit you as an individual in other ways than dieting, but larger than optimal amounts of vitamins for you will not increase your rate of fat-burning.

In *Supernutrition: Megavitamin Revolution*, which I wrote several years ago (Dial Press, 1975; Pocket Books, 1976), I showed how individuals could find the best levels of vitamins for themselves, and I am a proponent of taking vitamin and mineral supplements to help you reach your peak of health, not just achieving or maintaining average health. If I knew of evidence that more and more vitamins would help you lose weight, I would say so.

A B-COMPLEX SUPPLEMENT IS IMPORTANT

There is evidence that the B-Complex vitamins along with vitamin C helps the body deal with the stress of dieting. Also, many dieters have told me that extra amounts of the B-Complex vitamins plus vitamin C help keep their energy levels high and reduce emotional strains. Therefore, I recommend taking a B-Complex vitamin formula and vitamin C at dinner to replenish these water-soluble vitamins that leave the body in 6 to 8 hours after eating. The morning supplement, a general purpose multivitamin, multimineral capsule, provides what you need for the active part of the day, while the dinner supplement of the water-soluble B-Complex vitamins and vitamin C replenish your supply of what is lost quickly.

ACIDOPHILUS WILL HELP DIETERS

I do recommend taking *Lactobacillus Acidophilus* to maintain a significant level of this "good" bacterium in your intestine while your body is adjusting to a new diet. *L. Acidophilus* can help maintain regularity and your resistance to disease during the diet.

You can drink Acidophilus milk, which is a good source of *L. Acidophilus*, at your meals in place of skim milk, because it is skim milk with the bacterium added for your convenience. Acidophilus milk is available in many large supermarkets, health food stores, and of course, directly from dairies. Or you may prefer to take a daily acidophilus capsule, which is available from health food and drug stores.

TRY TO AVOID TAP WATER

The glasses of water that are required at meals and snacks would be more beneficial if the water were good *un*chlorinated spring, well, or mineral water, or even filtered through carbon-cartridge filters that can be attached to your faucet. Bottled mineral water is popular with joggers and is excellent for dieting.

Table 24.1 lists the required and recommended supplements for the Easy No-Flab Diet. Suggested strengths are given in Table 24.2. All supplements are available in all health food stores and in many drug stores and large supermarkets.

The supplements may be discontinued after the diet if desired. You may find increased health benefits from these supplements and wish to continue taking all or most of them regularly. They are wise investments in your health in these days of highly processed foods and widespread pollution.

TABLE 24-1
Supplements for the Easy No-Flab Diet

Supplement	Required	Strongly Recommended	Good Idea
Multiple vitamin–mineral	X		
B-Complex		X	
Calcium		X	
Lactobacillus Acidophilus		X	
Vitamin C		X	
Bran			X

TABLE 24-2
Suggested Strengths for Supplements

Multiple Vitamin–Mineral Pill (to be taken with breakfast)

Nutrient	Minimum Levels
Vitamin A, USP	10,000
Vitamin B-1, mg	25
Vitamin B-2, mg	25
Vitamin B-6, mg	25
Vitamin B-12, mcg	50
Niacinamide, mg	50
Choline, mg	25
Inositol, mg	25
Paba, mg	25
Pantothenic Acid, mg	50
Biotin, mcg	20
Folic Acid, mcg	100
Vitamin C, mg	150
Vitamin D, USP	100
Vitamin E, i.u.	50
Calcium, mg	25
Magnesium, mg	3
Zinc, mg	1
Potassium, mg	0.1
Iron, mg	5
Manganese, mg	1

TABLE 24-3
B-Complex Capsule

(Recommended to be taken at dinner)

Nutrient	Minimum Levels
B-1, mg	10
B-2, mg	10
B-6, mg	10
B-12, mcg	10
Niacinamide, mg	10
Choline, mg	10
Inositol, mg	10
Paba, mg	10
Pantothenic Acid, mg	25

ADDITIONAL

Vitamin C
250 to 1000 mg with dinner
Calcium
Either 500 mg calcium lactate or 100 mg of chelated calcium daily
Other Supplements
Bran: as package label suggests
Lactobacillus Acidophilus: as package label suggests

NO-FLAB EXERCISES— GETTING STARTED

25 EXERCISE MAY NOT BE YOUR FAVORITE recreation, but as you trim down, you may find yourself liking it better and better. It will speed up your fat-burning rate and at the same time shape your body to smooth out unwanted bulges.

Dieters are all in the same boat. No matter what shape we used to be in, we have to start all over again. A few years ago, we may have been able to whip off dozens of sit-ups and run for a mile, but now we may have to start with 1 or 2 sit-ups and walk the mile.

Coping with this reality may be the most frustrating part of your diet experience. But, if you follow the program, you will have control of your stomach (abdominal wall) muscles in just 2 weeks. And you will have a flat firm stomach in as few as 6 weeks, depending on how soon you get within 10 pounds of your desired weight.

CHECK WITH YOUR DOCTOR FIRST

No one should start a vigorous exercise program without checking with a physician. I recommend striding as an exercise rather than jogging, but **if you decide to jog rather than stride, be sure that when you call your physician to check on the diet program, you make an appointment for a *stress test*. No one over the age of 35 should start jogging without having a stress test.**

The stress test is an electrocardiogram taken while stepping up and down on a step, or stationary jogging on a conveyor belt. Some heart problems do not show up while the heart is at rest, and will only be revealed under exercise conditions. It's bothersome to go get a stress test, but you only live once. The stress test misses some potential heart problems, but it catches most of the serious problems. You want to lose fat, not your life.

TUMMY FLATTENERS

Start your exercise program tomorrow by doing a total of 10 sit-ups each day for the next 3 days. If you can do 10 consecutive sit-ups, fine; if you can't, do as many as you can, then rest a while and do some more.

If you have been doing sit-ups and can do more than 10, continue doing whatever you are used to.

If you can't do sit-ups right now, begin by doing reverse sit-ups and build your abdominal strength until you can do sit-ups. Reverse sit-ups are described in Note 25-1

NOTE 25-1
Exercises to Prepare You for Sit-Ups

A **reverse sit-up** is not a sit-down. Here's how it's done. Sit on the floor with your knees bent. Place your feet flat on the floor with your heels near your buttocks. Put your hands to the side and slightly behind you for support. Tuck your chin to your chest. Curve your back forward, reduce the support from your arms, and lower your back to the floor in an uncoiling motion.

Return to your original position by using your arms to raise your back. Repeat 4 more times. After a half hour or so, do 5 more reverse sit-ups.

On the second day, do 10 in the morning and 10 in the evening.

On the third day, do 10 in the morning, 10 in the afternoon, and 10 at night.

On the fourth day, advance to **tummy tighteners.** Sit on the floor with your knees bent, but this time straighten your back, move your feet forward, and spread your knees and feet several inches apart. Grasp your outer thighs (midthigh to near knee) keeping your elbows high and bent outward. Keep your back straight as you lower it until the small of your back touches the floor.

Now, let go of your legs and stretch your arms above your head. Hold this position for 6 to 10 full seconds. If your lower back rises off the floor when you let go of your legs, grab your thighs again a little higher and round your back. It is important that your lower back stay on the floor. Now let go of your legs, straighten your back, stretch your arms above your head, and hold for 6 to 10 seconds.

If you can't hold the hands-over-the-head position for 6 to 10 seconds at first, relax when it feels uncomfortable, rest a while, and start again.

As you lower your upper back, your abdominal muscles work harder. Do this exercise 3 times a day, working up to 10 repetitions in each set.

After working up to 3 sets of 10 repetitions each, try doing sit-ups again. Sit-ups should be easy by then, but if they're still hard to do, continue doing the tummy tighteners and try sit-ups from time to time.

A SPECIAL ISOMETRIC EXERCISE

Every time you complete a set of sit-ups, reverse sit-ups, or tummy tighteners, rest a moment or two and do the following isometric exercise.

An isometric exercise is one in which without any apparent motion, you control a muscle.

Sit erect on the floor with your legs extended in front of you. Take a deep breath, exhale fully to force the air out with a "whoosh," and before inhaling suck in your gut (draw in your stomach) as hard as you can for 6 to 10 seconds. Then relax, and repeat once again.

This effective exercise can be done a couple of times a day when you are seated, driving, riding, at a desk, watching TV, or standing. As you strengthen your abdominal wall, you can pull in your stomach so far that it will seem almost if you are making your belly button touch your spine. The important thing is that your tummy will be getting and staying flat.

THE EXERCISE FOR A PERMANENTLY TRIM TUMMY

As soon as you can do 10 consecutive sit-ups, start off each day with 10. Make this a lifetime habit; 10 little sit-ups every morning take less than a half minute, yet will keep your stomach flat. Even if you are thin, your stomach will bulge unless you maintain the abdominal wall strength.

I try to do 100 sit-ups a day, and often do more than 200. But many people will miss several days in a row because they can't find time. Eventually they may give up sit-ups altogether. While it's nice to do 100 or so every once in a while, it's more important to do 10 every day without exception. Don't consider skipping those 10 sit-ups any more than you would consider not eating.

Don't try to be a star and do 25 or 50 in the morning; just do those 10 every single morning (and then do others as you find time).

Maintain your new figure with as many sit-ups as you wish, but be sure to get those 10 sit-ups in every single day without exception. You can even do them without getting out of bed.

VARY YOUR SIT-UPS

Sit-ups are best done by bending your knees to make a 45° angle with the floor, to prevent back strain. On alternate days, you can do alternate styles of sit-ups for variety.

One day do the **arms extended sit-ups,** where you lie on your back with your arms extended back on the floor behind your head, and rise, with your back straight, to touch your toes. Raise and lower yourself slowly. It's easier to jerk, but that uses your hips and back more than your abdominal muscles.

On alternate days, do the **hands-behind-the-neck style.** Lie on your back with your hands behind your neck, your figners interlocked, elbows pointed forward. Smoothly, curl your back upward until your elbows touch your knees. Carefully curl your body as much as possible by moving your face as close to your abdomen as possible. Even if you can't raise up far, curl as much as possible.

Each style develops slightly different regions of the abdominal and back muscles (with considerable overlap). For both styles, it will help to lock your feet under heavy furniture.

WHEN IT'S TIME TO MOVE ON

After 2 weeks of 10-a-day sit-ups, add **leg raises** to strengthen your lower abdominal wall. There are two styles of leg raises. Just as you alternate sit-up styles, alternate leg-raise styles.

The first style is the **bent-knee raise,** in which you lie on your back, keep your arms behind your head, and grasp heavy furniture. Start with your legs together and fully extended on the floor. Raise your legs off the floor an inch or two and bend your knees to bring your heels up against your buttocks. Still keeping your legs off the floor, straighten and extend your legs to the starting position, only don't let your legs rest on the floor. Repeat for a 10-repetition total.

The second style of leg raise is to start from the same position, but keep your **knees locked** while lifting your legs straight up until they're perpendicular to the floor or as close as you can get. Then slowly lower your legs to the starting position, without letting them rest on the floor. Repeat for a total of 10 repetitions.

These tummy flatteners will not burn fat from around your stomach, but they will shrink your waistline and hold it in. You won't feel so fat while you are melting the fat away.

NOW IT'S TIME FOR PUSH-UPS

Another help in restoring your shape is to fill out the chest muscles in men and bustline in women by doing push-ups. Just 5 to 10 push-ups 3 or 4 times a week will bring good symmetry to your upper body. Most people can't do more than 2 or 3 to start with. If you can't do any, start with a **reverse push-up.** Support yourself at arm's length from the floor with your weight on your toes and hands and slowly lower your body to the floor while keeping your body straight. Climb back into the starting position and repeat again.

After you can do 10 repetitions of reverse push-ups, try doing a **modified push-up** in which you support your weight on your knees instead of your toes. Work your way up to 10 a day by increasing your number of repetitions 1 at a time every other day.

Then graduate to regular push-ups (toes on floor) and again work your way up to 10 by increasing one every two to three days, or as often as you can.

INCREASING BASAL METABOLISM TO SPEED FAT-BURNING

The tummy flatteners and push-ups will shape you, but you also need to step up your metabolism to increase your fat-burning process.

The increase in basal metabolism that occurs with regular exercise has been measured experimentally by Sports Medicine researchers, such as Dr. Dave Costill of Ball State University (Congress on Sports Medicine, Washington, D.C., May 1978). The effect is considerably more pronounced in men than in women.

The activity must last a sufficient amount of time so that the body stokes-up its energy production (by burning

213

fat) and must be regular enough so that the body keeps the energy production mechanism fully stoked.

If you make moderate energy demands on your body, it responds better by maintaining an improved state of readiness to make energy out of fat than if you make only rare energy demands on it.

You can increase the energy demand you place on your body to increase fat-burning rates through exercise. The objective is to begin slowly by stretching your muscles to reduce the chance of injury and then gradually increase your activity so that your respiration and pulse rates also gradually increase over a 5-minute period to your exercise rate.

If your physician approves after stress-testing you, you can test your condition by exercising at an activity level that raises your pulse by 20 to 30 beats a minute over your resting rate for a period of 12 minutes or until you're tired, whichever comes first.

You should exercise with a partner, particularly at first. **If at any time you feel chest pain *or pressure,* discontinue the exercise immediately and rest. If the pain or pressure subsides quickly, inform your physician of the occurrence as soon as you can get to a phone. If the pain or pressure doesn't disappear quickly, continue to rest, but as a precaution, ask your exercise partner to summon medical assistance.**

After exercising at the level that increased your pulse by 20 to 30 beats for 12 minutes, rest for 1 minute, and see if your pulse drops at least 10 counts per minute. If your pulse doesn't fall at least 10 counts 1 minute after exercising, do not exercise at this level, but drop to an activity level that increases your pulse by only 10 to 20 beats per minute for 12 minutes or until you're tired, whichever occurs first.

As the weeks pass, you can gradually increase your exercise rate as long as your pulse falls by 10 counts 1 minute after exercising.

TABLE 25-1

Ideal Exercising Pulse Rates for Healthy Persons (after gradual 5-minute warm-up). (Reprinted from *Supernutrition for Healthy Hearts*, Dial Press, 1977.)

Age	Ideal Exercise Pulse	Maximum Safe Rate
25	140–170	200
30	136–165	194
35	132–160	188
40	128–155	182
45	124–150	176
50	119–145	171
55	115–140	165
60	111–135	159
65	107–130	153
70	103–125	148
75	100–122	143
80	97–118	139
85	95–115	135
90	92–111	131
95	89–108	127
100	87–105	124

Ideal exercising rates for healthy individuals of various ages are given in Table 25-1. Once you are in shape enough to exercise at your ideal rate, you can now choose an exercise activity that will help you lose flab faster and also make you healthier. The next chapter explains how to have fun doing some pleasant activities such as walking, swimming, biking, dancing, or jogging, while getting the most benefit from them.

NO-FLAB EXERCISES—
WHEN YOU'RE IN SHAPE

26 A MODERATE LEVEL OF GENERAL DAILY activity is essential to good health. Bending, stretching, standing, walking, and climbing do more than burn calories. They stimulate muscle repair, improve circulation, muscle tone, and stimulate our internal organs.

Systematic exercising adds even further advantages. Exercising eases stress and tension, chases depression, improves sex, sleep, and resistance to disease, lowers blood-cholesterol levels, strengthens bones, helps you think better, rejuvenates, keeps you active longer, and leaves you with a general feeling of well-being and alertness for 10 to 12 hours afterwards.

Data from the American Cancer Society shows that the death rate of men between the ages of 45 and 65 who exercise regularly is 4 times lower than that of those who don't. Dr. Paul Metzer, Associate Medical Director for the Nationwide Insurance Company, says, "Just because you are past forty, don't think you're too old for regular exercise. Ten minutes of exercise will double the blood

216

level of adrenaline, which boosts your spirits and destroys depression."

NASA studies show that an exercise program can result in a lower resting heart rate, lower blood pressure, increased stamina, better feeling of well-being, reduced weight, and reduced stress and tension.

Your goal should be to get proper nourishment, exercise, and rest. All three are vital links in the fat-loss chain. It's a sign of middle age when all you exercise is caution.

WHY EXERCISE SHOULD BE REGULAR

Exercise is a magic potion, but it must be practiced at least 3 to 5 times a week. It is only the regularity of exercising that develops the enzymes that burn fat even while you're resting.

EXERCISE DOESN'T INCREASE APPETITE

That's right. A good workout doesn't make you hungrier than you would otherwise be. After 2 hours' tennis you may have "worked up an appetite," but that's because you didn't begin to play the minute you finished your last meal, and some time has passed since you've eaten.

Controlled studies by Dr. Lawrence B. Oscat (Associate Professor of Physical Education at the University of Illinois) have proven that exercise does *not* increase the appetite. He has found that 1 hour of exercise a day will not give you a desire to eat more food.

The appestat malfunctions if we don't maintain a certain activity level. So if you don't exercise, you may end up eating too much and become flabby rather than firm. Develop a sound body—not a round body.

THE BEST EXERCISE IS THE EXERCISE YOU ENJOY THE BEST

Exercise can be fun if you pick an activity you enjoy. With some people this may be a group or team sport, while others may wish solitude and privacy. Regardless of the activity you choose, it will only help burn calories. But if you are a little bit scientific about it, you can ensure that it will additionally develop the enzymes that will continue to burn fat even after you stop exercising. For most healthy people, this extra bonus comes from making sure that your pulse exceeds 120 beats per minute for 12 minutes every day, or for 20 minutes 5 days a week, or for 30 minutes 3 days a week.

I have found that some exercises are better for most people than others. Consider the following suggestions.

Striding—The Exercise for Nearly Everyone

Walking at a fast pace may not sound like the greatest exercise, but it is. Walking is the most efficient exercise and one that you can follow all the years of your life, or begin at any age or in almost any condition. Striding (walking briskly) improves blood circulation to improve each body cell's nourishment while preventing obesity.

Striding is safe, because the work load is smaller than during more strenuous exercises; thus the changes in your body physiology occur more slowly.

If a warning sign of too much exertion occurs while you're striding, such as tightness, pressure or pain in the chest, you will be able to notice it in plenty of time to reduce your exertion before serious harm occurs.

Jogging Is Fine for Active People

I love to jog, but jogging is a constant shock to the feet, and I occasionally injure an arch. Not everyone should

218

jog, nor should anyone over 35 jog without a stress test and a physician's okay.

Running is good for most active people, but as running becomes more popular, the fatalities mount. A U.S. congressman from the State of Maryland died while jogging in October, 1978. He had finished jogging 12 miles when he had his fatal heart attack. He had completed four Boston Marathons (26 miles and 385 yards) and had been a serious runner for more than 15 years. The message here is not that running killed him, as he may have died years earlier without running. The message is that running, by itself, doesn't protect you against heart disease, as so many believe. Also the message is that a person can get the benefits of running, with more safety, by striding.

Joggers run for pleasure and health benefits. You can find both in striding. But joggers tend to be competitive and will not easily stop before reaching a personal milepost or time goal. Joggers always seem to push farther. But when I stride, I lose the competitive compulsion and enjoy the brisk walk.

Distance Is More Important Than Speed

The distance covered in striding or jogging is more important than the speed. Running hard for 5 miles burns only 15 to 20 percent more calories than walking the same distance. The difference is even less if you take long strides, swing your arms, draw in your waist, and pull your chest up.

Striding is a pleasant habit, and one that can be shared with one or more companions. The ideal pace is that of a military march, covering about 3½ to 4 miles per hour. Of course, you don't have to walk a 3½-mile course—you can walk around and around the same block if you wish.

Striding at the 3½-miles per hour pace burns 5 calories a minute over your resting rate. **One hour a day of strid-**

ing will burn off 31 pounds in a year, not counting the calories burned because of your increased metabolic rate.

Get out and discover nature or your **real** neighborhood. Stride in all directions from your residence, once you're sure of the pace. Hum a march to help set the pace at first. Try for a minimum of 5 20-minute walks or 3 30-minute walks a week.

If you can't stride for a full 20 minutes, stride as far as you can comfortably and then continue at a slower pace until you have walked a total of 3 to 5 miles. You will probably be able to stride the full time in 2 to 4 weeks.

After 4 to 6 weeks of striding, you may even wish to add intervals of faster walking. Try it—you may like it.

If you're young and in good health, you might prefer to jog. If you are older and have been striding for a few months, you might also want to try jogging. But remember the increased risk and get medical approval first. If you want to try jogging, you may find the suggestions in Appendix II useful. They are from the President's Council on Physical Fitness and Sports.

Bad Weather Alternatives

In cold weather, I don't enjoy jogging or regular long walks as much, so I change my routine. This also helps me from getting bored and gives me a great desire to resume regular jogging or striding as spring nears.

In cold or rainy weather, I do cardio-pulls on an exercise apparatus. I also jump rope and do high kicks. Rheo Blair (nutritionist to the Stars) taught me that high kicks produce aerobic (cardiopulmonary) exercise and flatten the tummy as well. My wife is impressed with the ease of the high-kick exercise and the benefits of it. In the spring and summer she jogs, but in winter she, too, turns to high kicks.

The **high kick** is simple but amazingly effective. Just as striding is a form of marching, so is the high kick when you do a lot of repetitions.

Three to 5 minutes will do a lot for you, but you need to work longer than that. After you have done as many high kicks as you can, then jump rope, do knee bends, or aerobic exercises, such as the cardio-pulls or stepping up and down on a stair step.

Here is how Rheo Blair suggests doing high kicks:

Rise on the toes, then while keeping each leg straight—locked at the knee—KICK your right foot as high as you can, bring it down, and KICK your left foot as high as you can, alternating with each leg, and keep doing this until you are moderately tired.

In the beginning, 10 repetitions, which is 5 kicks with each leg, is probably enough for one set. Then, after you have rested a bit, you can do another set of 10 repetitions, which is 5 kicks with each leg. Rest a few minutes more, or you can even wait, and do another set of 10 repetitions, which is 5 kicks with each leg, just before you go to bed. As you become more conditioned, and as you become more flexible, you will find that you will be able to do more repetitions during each set.

Please take it easy at first! Remember, some of those muscles have not been used for years— and they will cry out to high heaven, poor things!

When you are able to do a hundred perfect high kicks, which is 50 repetitions with each leg, you will be in much better condition than you are now. You will also notice that the exercise stimulates breathing, and will definitely increase your endurance and lung power. You will find this an enjoyable exercise, it is most delightful. You will also find, after taking a warm bath or a shower, that it is much easier to kick even higher, as your muscles will be more supple.

STAYING TRIM

You don't have to stop here. You can do some more figure-shaping or body-strengthening if you like. There are many good books and courses available.

Tables 26-1 and 26-2 indicate the rate at which activities will burn calories. With the Easy No-Flab Diet the calories that are burned will be from fat. With the Easy No-Flab Diet, exercise, and more general activity, the flab will just drop off. You will look trim and lean.

You can take up tennis, golf, swimming, biking, soccer, dancing, or hiking. You may have a favorite sport you haven't played in years. Give it a try again, but start slowly. You may find yourself enjoying life more.

Whatever you do, you will feel better, look better, and like your new self better.

TABLE 26-1
Minutes of Activity Required to Burn
100, 200 or 300 Calories

	Minutes of Activity				
Calories	Striding	Walking	Biking	Jogging	Swimming
100	12	19	15	10	12
200	24	38	30	20	24
300*	36	57	45	30	36

* Suggested daily activity level

TABLE 26-2
Calories Consumed During Various Exercises
(Compiled by the National Frozen Food Association)

Job Activity	Calories Used Per Hour
Answering telephone	50
Bathing	100
Bed-making	300
Benchwork, sitting	75
Benchwork, standing	125
Bookkeeping	50
Brushing hair	100
Brushing teeth	100
Chopping a tree	480
Dictating	50
Dishwashing	75
Dressing, undressing	50
Driving tractor	150
Driving truck	100
Dusting furniture	150
Filing (office)	200
Gardening	250
Hammering (carpentry)	250
Hanging up wash	270
Ironing	100
Knitting	50
Laundering	200
Mopping floors	200
Mowing the lawn	460
Preparing food	100
Reading	25
Sawing	500
Scrubbing floors	200
Sewing	50
Shoveling	500
Sitting	70
Standing	80
Stoking a furnace	675

Job Activity	Calories Used Per Hour
Sweeping floors	150
Taking dictation	50
Telephoning	80
Typing	50
Walking upstairs and down	800
Washing your face	150
Writing	50

Recreation	Calories Used Per Hour
Badminton	400
Baseball	350
Basketball	550
Boating, rowing slow	400
Boating, rowing fast	800
Boating, motor	150
Bowling	250
Boxing	700
Calisthenics	500
Card playing	25
Croquet	250
Cycling, slowly	300
Cycling, strenuously	600
Dancing, slow step	350
Dancing, fast step	600
Driving a car	170
Field hockey	500
Fishing	150
Football	600
Golfing	250
Handball	550
Hiking	400
Horseback riding	250
Hunting	400
Jogging	600
Karate	600

Recreation	Calories Used Per Hour
Motorcycling	150
Painting	150
Piano playing	75
Running, fast-pace	900
Shuffleboard	250
Singing	50
Skating, leisurely	400
Skating, rapidly	600
Skiing	450
Soccer	650
Softball	350
Squash	550
Swimming, leisurely	400
Swimming, rapidly	800
Tennis, singles	450
Tennis, doubles	350
Volleyball	200
Walking, leisurely	200
Walking, fast	300
Watching television	25

THE EASY NO-FLAB MAINTENANCE DIET

27 BECOMING NATURALLY SLENDER IS A RE-warding experience. But don't slim down only to eat poorly again, because if you do, you'll start storing fat again in all those unattractive spots.

THE EASY NO-FLAB MAINTENANCE DIET

The good foods you eat during the Easy No-Flab Diet are the nucleus for a permanent No-Flab Maintenance Diet that will keep you naturally slender without effort. These good foods will nourish your body bringing better health and they'll help you live better longer. They'll give you a better figure and more energy for a more vivacious personality.

The Easy No-Flab Maintenance Diet will help you add high-quality foods to the Easy No-Flab Diet, until your weight stabilizes at your ideal weight. This process of stabilizing your weight will take about 3 to 4 weeks.

Many people make the mistake of getting their weight

down to their desired level and then switching to a normal diet before they have stabilized their weight. Switching to a normal diet too soon can jeopardize all the progress you've made, so it's best to take the Maintenance Diet as seriously as the Reducing Diet.

STABILIZING YOUR WEIGHT

Your appestat will reset itself for a diet that will maintain your desired weight automatically if you reset it properly. At the end of your dieting program your appestat will be adjusted at too low a level to maintain your ideal weight. If you suddenly splurge on sugary or empty-calorie (high insulin-release) foods, your blood-sugar level will begin the gyrations that will upset your appestat and cause gnawing hunger.

Slowly increasing the amount of good food you eat will bring the fat-loss process to a gradual halt without overshooting seriously. During this stabilization period you should weigh yourself every day. You should let your weight drop to about 2 pounds below the weight you wish to maintain, and then bring your weight up to the desired point at an average of a quarter pound per week.

Unfortunately, some people could continue to gain at a slight rate and not realize it until they have put on an extra 5 pounds. To avoid this, you should continue to chart your weight daily for 3 months after you have finished your fat-loss diet program. Then you should chart your weight on a weekly basis for a second 3-month period. From then on, you should weigh yourself weekly, although there will be no need to chart the weighings.

After you have maintained your desired weight for 2 or 3 weeks, you will not have to count FLAB Units or calories as long as you continue to eat those foods above 50 in the FLAB Index.

YOU CAN EAT A FEW SWEETS

Of course, you can have occasional cakes, cookies, or candies, without harm or upsetting your appestat. I would suggest that most people keep the amount of such foods that rank below 50 in the Flab Index to less than 2 percent of the weekly diet.

For example, if you are consuming 2,300 calories a day and maintaining your desired weight, first multiply your daily calorie intake by 7 to obtain your weekly calorie intake (7 × 2,300 = 16,100). Then take 2 percent of this total (16,100 × .02 = 322) to determine the number of calories a week of poorer quality food you can eat without gaining Flab.

Some individuals will be able to tolerate more low-quality food and others less. A 5 percent level has started many a person on the way to obesity.

If you eat junk in place of good food, your health will suffer, your hunger will increase—and you'll start putting on Flab. Again—empty calories mean full pounds.

HOW THE MAINTENANCE DIET WORKS

For the Maintenance Diet to work, you'll need to know how many FLAB Units you should eat each day. Because you'll no longer be losing Flab, the number of FLAB Units will be larger than while you were on the Reducing Diet. Begin by using Table 27-1 to find the number of calories you will need daily depending on your age and ideal weight. Then use Table 27-2 to find the number of FLAB Units and grams of protein you should include each day in your Maintenance Diet. Remember to spread the totals in generally equal thirds at breakfast, lunch, and dinner.

228

TABLE 27-1
The Calories You'll Need to Maintain Your Ideal Weight

(The approximate calorie needs for maintaining body weight for individuals who engage in light physical activity—adapted from Recommended Dietary Allowances, National Academy of Sciences)

Weight	Calorie Needs at Age		
	22	45	65
Women			
88	1,550	1,450	1,300
99	1,700	1,550	1,450
110	1,800	1,650	1,500
121	1,950	1,800	1,650
128	2,000	1,850	1,700
132	2,050	1,900	1,700
143	2,200	2,000	1,850
154	2,300	2,100	1,950
Men			
110	2,200	2,000	1,850
121	2,350	2,150	1,950
132	2,500	2,300	2,100
143	2,650	2,400	2,200
154	2,800	2,600	2,400
165	2,950	2,700	2,500
176	3,050	2,800	2,600
187	3,200	2,950	2,700
198	3,350	3,100	2,800
209	3,500	3,200	2,900
220	3,700	3,400	3,100

TABLE 27-2
The FLAB Units and Protein You'll Need to Maintain Your Ideal Weight

(This table will guide you in designing your No-Flab Maintenance Diet menus by allowing you to convert the calories you need to maintain your ideal weight into FLAB Units and protein needed for your maintenance diet.)

Calories	Maximum FLAB Units	Minimum Grams Protein
1,200	1,000	60
1,300	1,085	60
1,400	1,170	60
1,500	1,250	65
1,600	1,335	65
1,700	1,420	65
1,800	1,500	70
1,900	1,585	70
2,000	1,670	70
2,100	1,750	75
2,200	1,835	75
2,300	1,920	75
2,400	2,000	80
2,500	2,085	80
2,600	2,170	80
2,700	2,250	85
2,800	2,335	85
2,900	2,420	85
3,000	2,500	90
3,100	2,585	90
3,200	2,670	90
3,300	2,750	100
3,400	2,835	100
3,500	2,920	100
3,600	3,000	100

VARIETY IS THE SPICE
OF A MAINTENANCE DIET

Try to diversify your Maintenance Diet menus as much as possible. In fact, try to vary your daily diet for the rest of your life as much as possible, because it's healthful. Make a real effort each day to include:

two servings from the milk group
two servings from the meat group
four servings from the fruit/vegetable group
and
four servings from the grain group.
Single-serving equivalents of each group are listed below.*

---

*(Based on information of the National Dairy Council)

Milk Group

1 cup milk
1 cup yogurt
1 1/2 slices (1 1/2 oz) cheese
2 cups cottage cheese†

---

†Count cheese as serving of milk OR meat, not both simultaneously.

Meat Group

2 oz cooked lean meat, fish, poultry
2 eggs
2 slices (2 oz) cheese
1/2 cup cottage cheese*
1 cup dried beans, peas
4 tbsp peanut butter

---

*(Based on information of the National Dairy Council)

Fruit-Vegetable Group

1/2 cup juice
1/2 cup cooked
1 cup raw
Portion commonly served such as medium-sized apple or banana

Grain (whole grain) Group

1 sl bread, whole wheat or rye
1 cup ready-to-eat cereal, unsweetened
1/2 cup cooked cereal, pasta, grits

Don't forget your vitamin pills. If you stick with good nutrition, once out, that thin person inside you can stay out forever.

WHEN YOUR WEIGHT HAS STABILIZED

At this point my part is nearly done—I've suggested a safe and effective program to trim away and keep away Flab. Here's where your part becomes more important. You must supply the pride and desire not only to start the program but to stick with good foods after you reach your desired weight. It's easier to lose fat and keep it off than you may think—it gets easier when you gain control of your body chemistry.

TAKING IT OFF
AND KEEPING IT OFF

NOW YOU'RE AWARE THAT LOSING FAT is different from losing weight. You know you can eat more and weigh less. The Easy No-Flab Diet was designed to be easy. That's why it's so effective.

ONE STEP AT A TIME

Follow the Easy No-Flab Diet as a wise philosopher once advised we deal with a long journey—one step at a time. With the No-Flab Diet, take 1 pound off at a time. Each pound lost will offer a reason to be pleased and compliment yourself.

Don't worry about the entire 20 or 30 pounds you may want to lose. They will take care of themselves, if you take care of losing 1 pound at a time.

GETTING STARTED

Mark your progress as shown in Chapter 15, "Measuring Your Fat-loss." Progress will get easier and easier. But where will you be if you never start?

The first day is the hardest because you will have to remember to eat the snacks, and to say "no" to junk food.

By the third day, your habits will be fairly well established, and you'll be starting to burn fat without hunger.

Two weeks from now you will be able to measure significant improvements in blood pressure, cholesterol, triglycerides, and other parameters of health. I guarantee that you will lose fat healthfully while improving your nutrition.

That's all there is to it. Now turn to Chapter 17 "Starting Your Diet" and start your three-day countdown to a new and improved you.

This diet will work for you even if others have failed. Give it a chance and it will give you a new body, new vigor, and new health. Best Wishes and Good Health!

APPENDIX I

I. THE IDEAL REDUCING DIET

THE OPTIMAL PERCENTAGES IN THE DIET of protein, carbohydrates, and fat depend on the individual. Reasonable limits for a healthy diet for people of ideal weight would be protein 12 to 60 percent; fat 20 to 30 percent; and carbohydrate 20 to 68 percent.

The U.S. Department of Agriculture (USDA) figures show that the average daily diet of Americans from 1970 to 1976 was 15.7 percent protein, 24.5 percent fat, and 59.6 percent carbohydrates to provide a daily total of 3,300 calories (*BioScience*, March 1978). The following chart reveals their findings.

Average American Diet

Food Component	Grams	Cal	% Diet Wt	% Diet Cals
Protein	100	400	15.7	12
Fats	156	1,404	24.5	42
Complex Carbohydrates	181	716	28.4	22
Simple Carbohydrates	199	780	31.2	24
Total	636	3,300	99.8	100

An analysis of the data indicates that convenience foods are probably adding too many calories to America's diet. The main culprits in convenience foods are the increased use of vegetable oils and sugars, which add calories and upset the blood sugar level. Dr. George W. Kramer of USDA has said, "The mounting use of vegetable oils is the main reason why U.S. diets are richer in nutrient fats." (*Journal of the American Medical Association* November 21 1977)

THE IDEAL REDUCING DIET

A properly designed reducing diet would incorporate the following considerations:

1. The diet should include enough protein for body repair and maintenance of a good mood, but not too much so as to aggravate gout. The 100 gm of protein in the present American diet meets these requirements.

2. Enough complex carbohydrate should be provided for energy and to prevent ketosis (the acid blood caused by the incomplete burning of fat), but not so much simple carbohydrate as to stimulate hunger and stop fat-burning. The proportion of complex carbohydrate should exceed 65 percent of the total carbohydrate intake, and the simple carbohydrate should be only natural unrefined fruit or milk sugars in whole foods. Approximately 100 gm of carbohydrate will fulfill these requirements.

3. Sufficient fat should be included to ensure absorption of the fat-soluble vitamins and to promote healthy skin, hair, and nerves. Satiety can be achieved with 40 gm of fat daily.

The ideal reducing diet would include the following components:

	Gram	Cals	% Diet Wt	% Diet Cals
Protein	105	420	42	35
Fats	40	360	16	30
Complex Carbohydrates	69	276	28	23
Simple Carbohydrates	36	144	14	12
Total	250	1,200	100	100

The ideal reducing diet compares to the standard American diet as follows:

	Protein		Fat		Carbohydrate	
	Grams	% Cals	Grams	% Cals	Grams	% Cals
American Diet	100	12	156	42	380	46
Ideal Reducing	105	35	40	30	105	35

Note the reduction of fat and carbohydrate in the perfect reducing diet. Even though the percentages do not seem to change that drastically, the total quantity of each differs markedly due to the total food-quantity (calorie) reduction.

Keep in mind that the weights and percentages alone are meaningless, because a diet consisting of skin (protein), sugar (carbohydrate), and butter (fat) would result in death. The *quality* of the food is more important than the proportions of proteins, carbohydrates, and fats. The Easy No-Flab Diet excludes poor-quality foods from the diet and speeds fat-burning, while maintaining all of the advantages of the perfect reducing diets discussed above.

APPENDIX II

II. ADVANCED NO-FLAB
EXERCISES—JOGGING, INTERVAL
TRAINING, AND WARM-UP EXERCISES

MANY OF YOU MAY BE EXPERIENCED JOG-
gers who are steadily losing weight but wish to
safely speed up that rate by the Easy No-Flab
Diet. Others have progressed from the beginning exercises
and wish to jog rather than stride. If this includes you, and
you are in the shape discussed in Chapter 26 with a good
recovery rate of your pulse after vigorous exercise, and you
have had a stress test if you are over 35, then by all means
jog if you so wish.

Millions of people are jogging these days, and it seems to
come naturally. However, the following advice from the
President's Council on Physical Fitness and Sports should
be followed:

> Run in an upright position with your back
> straight and your head up. Avoid looking at your
> feet. Arms should be held slightly away from the
> body, with arms bent at the elbows and forearms
> parallel to the ground. To reduce the tightness
> that sometimes results while jogging, occasion-
> ally shake and relax your shoulders. Try to land

on the heel of the foot and rock forward so that you drive off the ball of the foot for your next step. Keep steps short (to reduce extension-type injuries) and breathe deeply with your mouth open. Don't hold your breath. If you become overly tired or uncomfortable, slow down, walk, or stop completely.

Clothes should be loose and comfortable. Avoid garments that restrict freedom of movement or impede blood circulation. Don't wear rubberized or plastic clothing. Increased sweating will not produce a permanent weight-loss and such clothing can cause body temperatures to rise and fall at dangerous levels. It also interferes with the evaporation of sweat. If sweat can't evaporate, heat stroke or heat exhaustion is a possibility. Wear shoes that fit properly and have firm soles, good arch supports, and pliable tops. (Jogging shoes are designed to prevent injuries and are an excellent investment.) Clean, heavy, soft socks should be worn at all times.

The actual time of day you jog isn't too important although studies indicate that people who jog early in the morning tend to follow a schedule better than those who jog in the evening. However, avoid jogging the first hour after eating or during the middle of a hot, humid day.

Running on tracks and grassy fields is most recommended, but any place will do. Try to avoid hard running surfaces such as concrete and asphalt for the first few weeks. Varying jogging routes and locations will add interest to your program. Jog alone or with a friend, but remember companionship—not competition—should be your goal here.

This personal jogging schedule may be used as a general guideline in beginning your running program. Just as with any kind of exercise, you may want to vary from the recommendations, depending on how you feel. The important thing is to jog regularly and progress at a comfortable rate.

SCHEDULE FOR BEGINNING JOGGERS
(President's Council on Fitness and Sports)

Week	Activity
1	Jog 40 sec (100 yds). Walk 1 min (100 yds). Repeat 9 times during each session [I recommend three alternate days a week for each activity].
2	Jog 1 min (150 yds). Walk 1 min (100 yds). Repeat 8 times.
3	Jog 2 min (300 yds). Walk 1 min (100 yds). Repeat 6 times.
4	Jog 4 min (600 yds). Walk 1 min (100 yds). Repeat 4 times.
5	Jog 6 min (900 yds). Walk 1 min (100 yds). Repeat 3 times.
6	Jog 8 min (1,200 yds). Walk 2 min (200 yds). Repeat 2 times.
7	Jog 10 min (1,500 yds). Walk 2 min (200 yds). Repeat 2 times.
8	Jog 12 min (1,700 yds). Walk 2 min (200 yds). Repeat 2 times.

INTERVAL TRAINING—THE PUFF AND REST METHOD

Many people prefer "Interval Training" to continuous exercising, especially when the exercise is running. Interval training is simply repeated periods of vigorous physical activity such as running, swimming, biking, etc., interspersed with recovery periods. Recovery periods are intervals of reduced exercise intensity (not complete rest) during which the heart, lungs, and muscles are allowed to recuperate without actually returning to a resting state.

If running is the activity you choose, run a specified time (such as 30 seconds), then jog or walk for an equal time. Repeat this procedure a number of times, depending on your condition, ability, and time available.

One form of interval training is "stutter" jogging—jogging 30 seconds, walking 30 seconds, and so on. Dr. M. L. Rendle of New Zealand studied two matched groups of unfit, middle-aged men. One group jogged four or five mornings weekly for 5 months; the other group stutter-jogged for the same amount of time. The stutter-joggers lost more flabby tissue than the straight joggers, and their general health improved equally as much.

Whenever you exercise, you should monitor your pulse and respiration. **If your pulse exceeds the suggested rate in Table 25-1** *or if your breathing becomes so labored that you can't carry on a conversation,* **you are pushing too hard** and should slow down. The President's Council on Physical Fitness and Sports recommends interval training as safe and effective.

WARMING UP AND COOLING DOWN

Your training period should be preceded by a warm-up of about 5 to 10 minutes—some preliminary bending, stretching, and running in place. The warm-up will guard your heart and circulatory systems from being suddenly overtaxed. And it will help keep your joints and muscles from becoming sore or injured.

A 5- to 10-minute cool-down period of reduced activity after your workout lets your system return to a pre-stress condition gradually—the best way. Don't start in "cold." And don't exercise and then stop "cold."

WARM-UP EXERCISES

It's important to do warm-up exercises before you start jogging or interval training. Do 1 exercise from each of the following groups.

Back-Stretching Group

Bend and Stretch—Stand straight with your feet shoulder-width apart. Bend your trunk forward and down, allowing your knees to bend. Gently stretch and extend your fingers to your toes or the floor. Return to your starting position. Don't stretch too much on the first try. Gradually increase the stretch.

Sitting Stretch—Sit with your legs spread far apart and hands on knees. Bend forward at the waist reaching your fingers as far forward down each leg simultaneously as you can with reasonable comfort. Return to your starting position and do the exercise again several times.

Toe Touch—Stand with your feet together. Bend your trunk forward and down, allowing a slight knee bend. With a light bouncing motion, reach lower and lower until your fingers touch your toes (or as close as you can get). Return to your starting position and do the exercise several times more. Alternate by stretching to one side and then to the other.

Trunk-Twisting Group

Body Twist—Stand with your feet shoulder-width apart and your arms extended outward from your sides, parallel to the floor. Twist your upper body as far as possible with reasonable comfort to each side, trying to gradually turn farther. Turn your neck at the same time.

Body Bend—Stand with your feet shoulder-width apart and your hands behind your neck with fingers interlaced. Raise your left knee above waist height while twisting your trunk to the left and bending so that your right elbow touches your left knee. Return to your starting position and repeat with your right knee and left elbow. Keep your fingers interlaced behind your neck. Do the exercise again, several times on each side.

Hamstring-Stretching Group

Dancer's Stretch—Stand in front of a flight of stairs or piece of furniture with a waist-high platform. Place one of your heels on the waist-high stair or platform with your toe pointed up. Straighten your leg and bend forward at the waist toward your extended leg. Gently rock to stretch the hamstring. Repeat with your other leg. You only need to do this exercise once with each leg.

Skier's Stretch—Stand 2 to 3 feet from a wall with your feet together. Touch the wall with your palms and lean toward the wall by bending your arms, all the while keeping your feet flat on the floor. If you don't feel any pull in the back of your calf muscles, move farther from the wall and try the exercise again. Three or four good stretches should do the job.

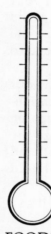

APPENDIX III

III. FOOD TABLES—FLAB UNITS, CALORIES
AND FLAB INDEX OF COMMONLY USED
FOODS

FOODS ARE LISTED UNDER THE FOLLOWING
CATEGORIES:
Milk Products
Meats and Other Protein-rich Foods
Fruits
Vegetables
Grain Products
Combinations
Miscellaneous

MILK PRODUCTS

Food	Serving Size	FLABs	Prote(gm)	Carbo(gm)	Fat(gm)	Cals	FLAB Index
Butter	1 tsp	36	tr*	tr	4.1	36	62.0
Buttermilk	1 cup	69	8.8	12.5	0.2	88	79.1
Cheese:							
American	1 oz (1 sl)	92	6.0	1.6	8.2	104	70.1
Blue	1 oz	97	6.0	1.0	9.0	105	67.1
Cheddar	1 oz	99	6.9	0.6	9.2	113	70.8
Cottage	1 oz	88	15.4	3.3	4.8	120	84.5
Muenster	1 oz	91	6.2	0.6	8.5	102	69.5
Roquefort	1 oz	97	6.0	1.0	9.0	105	67.1
Swiss	1 oz	87	8.0	0.5	7.7	103	73.4
Cream:							
Light	1 tbsp	29	tr	1.0	3.0	30	64.1
Sour	1 tbsp	22	tr	1.0	2.0	25	70.5
Whipped	1 tbsp	26	0.2	0.2	2.8	26	62.0
Half and Half	1 tbsp	20	0.5	0.7	1.8	20	62.0
Ice cream:							
Chocolate	1/2 cup	197	2.7	14.0	8.4	140	44.0
Vanilla	1/2 cup	190	2.7	13.7	8.3	138	45.0
Ice milk:							
Vanilla	1/2 cup	142	3.1	17.0	4.0	110	48.0

245

Food	Serving Size	FLABs	Prote(gm)	Carbo(gm)	Fat(gm)	Cals	FLAB Index
Milk, chocolate	1 cup	234	8.5	27.5	8.5	213	56.4
Milk, low-fat (2%)	1 cup	104	7.3	11.3	4.9	118	70.3
Milk, skim	1 cup	62	7.3	11.3	0.2	77	77.0
Milk, skim	3/4 cup	46	5.5	8.4	0.2	58	77.0
Milk, whole	1 cup	131	7.3	11.3	7.9	145	68.6
Milk, whole	3/4 cup	98	5.5	8.5	5.9	109	68.6
Milk, whole	1/2 cup	65	3.7	5.7	4.0	72	68.6
Milkshake:							
Chocolate	1 1/2 cup	507	12.1	49.5	17.6	391	47.8
Vanilla	1 1/2 cup	487	12.0	48.0	18.0	378	48.1
Yogurt:							
Plain	1 cup	110	11.5	15.0	2.9	130	73.3
Strawberry	1 cup	206	9.2	42.0	2.2	225	67.7
Vanilla	1 cup	179	9.9	33.8	2.8	200	69.1

* tr = trace (present, but too small to measure).

246

MEAT, FISH, AND OTHER PROTEIN-RICH FOODS

Food	Serving Size	FLABs	Prote(gm)	Carbo(gm)	Fat(gm)	Cals	FLAB Index
Almonds	1 cup	724	26.0	28.0	77.0	850	72.8
Bacon (nitrite-free)	1/2 oz (2 sl)	87	4.6	0.5	7.8	92	65.6
Beans, refried	1/2 cup	138	8.9	26.2	0.9	142	63.8
Beef:							
Ground	3 oz	133	23.3	0	9.6	186	86.7
Liver	3 oz	144	22.5	4.5	9.0	195	84.0
Sirloin steak	3 oz	130	22.0	0	9.5	180	85.8
T-Bone steak	3 1/2 oz	146	29.0	0	9.8	212	90.0
Top round	3 oz	169	24.6	0	13.3	225	82.5
Bologna	1 oz	81	3.4	0.3	7.8	86	65.8
Brazil nuts	1 cup	777	20.0	15.0	94.0	915	73.0
Cashew nuts	1 cup	736	23.0	40.0	62.0	760	64.0
Chicken:							
Fried	3 oz (leg & thigh)	142	26.0	1.6	9.3	201	87.8
Liver	1 oz	48	7.5	1.5	3.4	65	84.0
Broiled or Roasted	4 oz	138	35.2	0	7.5	218	97.9
Egg:							
Boiled	1 lrg	67	6.5	0.5	5.8	82	75.9

Food	Serving Size	FLABs	Prote(gm)	Carbo(gm)	Fat (gm)	Cals	FLAB Index
Fried	1 lrg	92	6.9	0.2	8.6	108	72.8
Scrambled	1 lrg	95	7.2	1.5	8.3	111	72.4
Fish:							
Breaded	3 oz	157	16.2	5.8	11.3	193	76.8
Broiled:							
Bluefish	3 oz	76	22.0	0	4.0	124	100.0
Flounder	3 oz	49	20.0	0	1.0	85	100.0
Haddock	3 oz	69	17.0	0	5.0	113	100.0
Mackerel	3 oz	110	19.0	0	13.0	193	100.0
Perch	3 oz	99	16.0	0	11.0	163	100.0
Red Snapper	5 oz	100	41.6	0	1.9	195	100.0
Shad	3 oz	95	20.0	0	10.0	170	100.0
Swordfish	3 oz	85	24.0	0	5.0	141	100.0
Canned:							
Salmon	3 oz	75	17.0	0	5.0	113	93.4
Sardines	(1/2 of 3 3/4 can)	74	11.0	0	8.0	115	96.4
Tuna	3 oz (1/2 cup)	112	24.5	0	7.0	168	93.0
Fish sticks	3 oz	157	16.2	5.8	11.3	193	76.8
Frankfurter (nitrite-free)	2 oz	146	7.0	0.9	15.4	172	73.0
Ham, baked (nitrite-free)	3 oz	121	25.7	0	7.7	179	91.7

Hamburger	3 oz	133	23.3	0	9.6	186	86.7
Lamb chop	3 oz	196	21.4	0	17.0	242	76.6
Meat loaf	3 oz	195	15.8	12.6	12.4	230	73.1
Meat patty (beef)	3 oz	133	23.3	0	9.6	186	86.7
Peanut butter	2 tbsp	191	8.9	5.5	15.8	186	60.4
Peanuts, unsalted	1/4 cup	181	9.4	6.8	17.9	211	72.3
Peas, blackeye:							
immature	1/2 cup	123	10.0	22.4	1.0	134	67.5
mature	1/2 cup	91	6.3	17.1	0.4	94	64.0
Pecans	1/4 cup	180	2.5	4.0	19.3	185	64.0
Pork chop, broiled	3 oz	255	20.8	0	24.2	308	74.9
Protein powder	1 oz	57	28.4	0	0	114	100.0
Sardines (see Fish, canned)							
Sausage	1 oz (2 links)	123	5.1	tr	12.5	135	77.5
Sirloin steak (see Beef)							
T-bone steak (see Beef)							
Top round steak (see Beef)							
Tuna (See Fish, canned)							
Turkey, Roasted or							
Broiled	4 oz	157	37.2	0	9.2	240	94.8
Veal, loin chop,							
Baked	3 1/2 oz	135	35.8	0	7.0	217	99.7

FRUITS

Food	Serving Size	FLABs	Prote(gm)	Carbo(gm)	Fat(gm)	Cals	FLAB Index
Apple	1 med	71	0.3	20.0	0.8	80	69.9
Apple juice	1/2 cup	60	tr	15.0	tr	60	62.0
Apple sauce	1/2 cup	134	0.3	30.4	0.1	116	53.7
Apricots, dried	4 halves	37	0.8	10.0	0.1	39	65.4
Avocado	1/2 med.	181	2.0	6.0	18.0	185	63.4
Banana	1 med.	111	1.3	26.4	0.2	114	63.7
Blueberries	1/2 cup	42	0.5	10.5	0.5	42	62.0
Cantaloupe	1/4 med.	29	0.7	7.2	0.1	29	62.0
Cherries	1/2 cup	40	1.0	10.0	0.1	40	62.0
Cranberry juice	1/2 cup	80	0.1	20.0	0.1	80	62.0
Cranberry sauce	1/2 cup	231	0.1	52.0	0.5	203	54.5
Dates	1/2 cup	245	2.0	65.0	0.5	245	62.0
Fig, dried	1 lrg	60	0.5	7.5	0.1	60	62.0
Fruit salad	1/2 cup	96	1.5	24.8	0.5	110	71.2
Fruit cocktail	1/2 cup	111	0.5	25.0	0.5	97	54.2
Grapefruit	1/2 med.	48	0.6	12.5	0.1	48	62.0
Grapefruit juice	1/2 cup	47	0.5	11.5	0.1	48	63.0
Grapes (all American types)	1/2 cup	48	0.4	12.3	0.2	48	62.0
Grape juice	1/2 cup	83	0.5	21.0	0.1	83	62.0
Lemon	1 med.	20	1.0	6.0	0.1	20	62.0

Food	Measure						
Lemon juice	1/2 cup	29	0.5	10.0	0.1	30	64.1
Lemonade	1/2 cup	79	0.1	14.0	0.1	55	43.2
Lime juice	1/2 cup	32	0.5	11.0	0.1	33	63.9
Nuts (see meats)							
Olive	4 med.	15	0.1	0.1	2.0	15	62.0
Orange	1 med.	61	1.3	16.0	0.3	65	66.1
Orange juice	1/2 cup	57	0.9	13.3	0.1	58	63.1
Papayas, cubed	1/2 cup	35	0.5	9.0	0.1	35	62.0
Peaches	1/2 cup	98	0.5	26.0	0.1	100	63.3
Pear	1 med.	100	1.2	25.3	0.7	101	62.6
Pineapple, diced	1/2 cup	36	0.5	9.5	0.1	38	65.4
Pineapple (water-pac) sliced ring	1 lrg	89	0.4	23.7	0.1	90	62.7
Pineapple juice	1/2 cup	68	0.5	17.0	0.1	68	62.0
Plum	1 med.	25	0.1	7.0	0.1	25	62.0
Prunes, stewed	4 med.	98	0.7	28.3	0.1	108	68.3
Raisins	4 1/2 tbsp	131	0.1	32.9	0.1	123	58.2
Raspberries	1/2 cup	35	0.5	8.5	0.5	35	62.0
Rhubarb, cooked, sweetened	1/2 cup	208	0.5	49.0	0.1	193	57.5
Strawberries	1/2 cup	28	0.5	6.3	0.4	28	62.0
Tangerine	1 med.	20	0.5	5.0	0.1	20	62.0
Watermelon	1 cup	52	1.0	12.8	0.4	52	62.0

VEGETABLES

Food	Serving Size	FLABs	Prote(gm)	Carbo(gm)	Fat(gm)	Cals	FLAB Index
Asparagus	4 spears (1/2cup)	11	1.3	2.2	0.1	12	67.3
Beans, baked (with pork and tomato sauce)	1/2 cup	148	7.8	24.2	3.3	156	65.4
Beans, green	1/2 cup	15	1.0	3.4	0.1	16	66.1
Beans, lima	1/2 cup	89	6.5	16.8	0.4	94	65.5
Beans, refried	1/2 cup	138	8.9	26.2	0.9	142	63.8
Beets	1/2 cup	30	0.8	7.3	0.1	31	64.1
Broccoli	1 stalk (1/2 cup)	23	2.4	3.5	0.2	26	70.1
Cabbage	1/6 hd (1/2 cup)	8	0.7	2.9	0.2	13	100.0
Carrots, cooked	1/2 cup	18	0.7	5.1	0.1	22	75.8
Carrot stick, raw	5″	13	0.6	4.9	0.1	21	100.0
Cauliflower	1/2 cup	12	1.4	2.5	0.1	13	67.2
Celery stick	8″ stalk	2	0.5	2.2	0.1	10	100.0
Coleslaw (with mayonnaise)	1/2 cup	76	0.7	2.7	7.9	82	66.9
Collards, cooked	1/2 cup	24	2.5	4.5	0.5	27	69.8
Corn, canned	1/2 cup	54	2.2	16.4	0.7	70	80.4
Corn, ear	5″ × 1 3/4″	87	4.1	26.3	1.3	114	81.2
Corn, flakes	3/4 cup	62	1.5	16.0	0.1	72	72.0
Corn, grits	1/2 cup	59	1.5	13.5	0.1	62	65.2
Corn, pop, plain	1 cup	9	0.8	4.6	0.3	23	100.0

Endive	1 oz	2	0.5	1.0	0.1	5	100.0
Greens	1/2 cup	15	1.9	2.9	0.2	17	70.3
Kale	1/2 cup	6	2.0	2.0	0.5	15	100.0
Lettuce (Boston)	1/6 hd	2	0.4	1.1	tr	5	100.0
Lettuce (iceberg)	1/6 hd (1/2 cup)	4	0.7	2.2	0.1	10	100.0
Lettuce (loose-leaf)	2 lrg	4	0.7	1.8	0.2	9	100.0
Okra	4 pods (1/2 cup)	10	0.9	2.6	0.1	12	74.4
Onions	1/2 cup	24	1.3	6.8	0.1	30	77.5
Parsley	1 tbsp	tr	tr	tr	tr	1	100.0
Parsnips	1/2 cup	45	1.0	11.5	0.5	50	68.9
Peas, blackeye (immature)	1/2 cup	123	10.0	22.4	1.0	134	67.5
(mature)	1/2 cup	91	6.3	17.1	0.4	94	64.0
Peas, green	1/2 cup	52	4.1	9.4	0.2	54	64.4
Pepper, green	1/4 lrg	5	0.3	1.2	0.5	5	62.0
Popcorn, plain	1 cup	9	0.8	4.6	0.3	23	100.0
Potato, baked	1 lrg	123	3.7	29.9	0.1	140	70.6
Potato, boiled	2 small	72	2.3	17.7	0.1	81	69.8
Potato chips	10	126	1.1	10.0	8.0	114	56.1
Potato, french-fried	20 (3 oz)	237	3.7	30.6	11.2	233	61.0
Potato, hash browns	1 oz	51	1.2	10.2	0.7	52	63.2
Potato, mashed	1/2 cup	63	2.0	12.7	0.7	74	72.8
Potato, sweet	1/2 med	68	1.2	17.9	0.3	78	71.1
Radishes	4 med	2	0.1	1.0	0.1	5	100.0
Salad, tossed	3/4 cup	7	0.7	2.7	0.1	13	100.0
Sprouts							
Mung bean	1/2 cup	11	1.5	3.0	0.1	15	84.5

Food	Serving Size	FLABs	Prote(gm)	Carbo(gm)	Fat(gm)	Cals	FLAB Index
Soy bean	1/2 cup	12	3.0	2.0	1.0	20	100.0
Squash, summer	1/2 cup	15	1.1	3.3	0.2	16	66.1
Squash, winter	1/2 cup (1/2 med.)	53	1.9	14.4	0.1	56	65.5
Sweet potato	1/2 med.	68	1.2	17.9	0.3	78	71.1
Tomato	1/2 med.	22	1.1	4.7	0.2	22	62.0
Tomato juice	1/2 cup	25	1.1	5.2	0.1	26	64.5
Tomato soup, creamed	1 cup	173	6.5	22.5	7.0	173	62.0
Tossed salad	3/4 cup	7	0.7	2.7	0.1	13	100.0
Turnips	1/2 cup	13	1.5	2.5	0.1	15	71.5
Vegetable juice	1/2 cup	25	1.1	5.2	0.1	26	64.5
Zucchini	1/2 cup	12	1.0	2.5	0.1	12	62.0

GRAIN PRODUCTS

Food	Serving Size	FLABs	Prote(gm)	Carbo(gm)	Fat(gm)	Cals	FLAB Index
Bagel	3" dia.	204	6.0	28.0	2.0	165	50.1
Biscuit	2" dia.	126	2.1	12.8	4.8	103	50.7
Bran flakes	1/2 cup	62	1.3	14.2	0.1	64	64.0
Bread, corn	2 1/2" × 3"	182	6.0	29.5	5.1	191	65.1
Bread, Italian	1 sl	59	2.0	12.8	0.2	63	66.2
Bread, rye	1 sl	51	2.0	11.8	0.2	55	66.9
Bread, white	1 sl	73	2.0	11.5	0.7	61	51.8
Bread, whole wheat	1 sl	51	2.4	10.8	0.7	55	66.9
Cereal (see specific grain)							
Corn bread	2 1/2" × 3"	183	6.0	29.5	5.1	191	65.1
Corn flakes	3/4 cup	62	1.5	16.0	0.1	72	72.0
Crackers, graham	2	77	1.1	10.3	1.3	54	43.5
Crackers, saltine	5	78	1.2	9.8	1.7	60	47.7
Grits, hominy	1/2 cup	59	1.5	13.5	0.1	62	65.2
Macaroni	1 cup	445	18.0	44.0	24.0	470	65.5
Noodles, egg	1/2 cup	95	3.3	18.6	1.2	100	65.3
Oatmeal	1/2 cup	64	2.4	11.6	1.2	66	63.9
Pancake	4" dia.	59	1.9	8.8	2.0	61	64.1
Rice	1/2 cup	106	2.1	24.8	0.1	112	65.5
Roll, frankfurter	1	136	3.3	21.2	2.2	119	54.2

Food	Serving Size	FLABs	Prote(gm)	Carbo(gm)	Fat (gm)	Cals	FLAB Index
Roll, hamburger	1	136	3.3	21.2	2.2	119	54.2
Roll, hard	1	178	4.9	29.8	1.6	156	54.2
Spaghetti	1 cup	151	5.0	32.0	1.0	155	63.6
Tortilla, corn	6" dia.	56	1.5	13.5	0.6	63	69.8
Waffles	2	122	4.2	17.1	5.0	130	66.1
Wheat flakes	2/3 cup	60	1.9	13.6	0.1	65	67.2
Wheat, puffed cereal	1 cup	49	2.3	11.8	0.2	54	68.0
Wheat, shredded	1 oz	91	3.0	23.0	1.0	100	68.1

COMBINATIONS

Food	Serving Size	FLABs	Prote(gm)	Carbo(gm)	Fat (gm)	Cals	FLAB Index
Beans, baked, with Pork and Tomato sauce	1/2 cup	148	7.8	24.2	3.3	156	65.4
Beef and vegetable stew	1 cup	179	15.0	14.6	10.1	209	72.4
Chef's salad (see No-Flab Lunch #9)		281	39.5	17.1	14.9	342	75.5
Chili con carne with beans	1 cup	308	18.8	30.5	15.3	333	67.0
Custard, baked	1/2 cup	144	7.2	14.7	7.3	152	65.4
Macaroni and cheese	1/2 cup	201	7.2	14.7	7.3	152	65.4
Pizza, cheese	1/4 of 14"	328	18.0	42.5	12.5	354	66.9
Sandwich, chicken salad	1	262	33.5	23.0	13.0	329	77.9
Sandwich, grilled cheese	1	268	16.8	24.8	17.8	318	73.6
Sandwich, ham & cheese	1	186	17.4	21.9	7.8	221	74.9
Sandwich, Pastrami	1	226	8.8	28.6	10.4	240	65.8
Sandwich, roast beef	1	184	21.8	21.6	6.8	231	77.8
Sandwich, tuna fish salad	1	275	24.6	24.7	15.1	332	74.9
Soup, chicken noodle	1 cup	55	3.2	7.5	1.8	59	66.5
Soup, cream of tomato	1 cup	173	6.5	22.5	7.0	173	62.0
Spaghetti, meatballs & tomato sauce	1 cup	308	18.6	38.7	11.7	332	66.8
Stew, beef & vegetable	1 cup	179	15.0	14.6	10.1	209	72.4
Taco, beef	1	183	16.9	14.7	10.0	216	73.2

MISCELLANEOUS

Food	Serving Size	FLABs	Prote(gm)	Carbo(gm)	Fat(gm)	Cals	FLAB Index
Alcoholic, cocktail (1 1/2 oz spirits in 10 oz cocktail)		146	0	tr	0	97	41.2
Bagel	3" dia.	204	6.0	28.0	2.0	165	50.1
Bar, candy	1 oz	285	2.2	16.1	9.2	147	32.2
Beer	1 1/2 cup	172	1.1	13.7	0	151	54.4
Cake, devil's food	1/16 of 9"	407	3.0	40.2	8.5	234	35.6
Cake, sponge	1/12 of 10"	335	5.0	35.7	3.8	196	36.3
Candy bar	1 oz	285	2.2	16.1	9.2	147	32.2
Cheesecake	4 oz or 1/6 of 8"	306	10.2	23.0	9.0	214	43.4
Cocktail (see Alcoholic, cocktail)							
Chocolate candy bar	1 oz	285	2.2	16.1	9.2	147	32.2
Chocolate milk	1 cup	234	8.5	27.5	8.5	213	56.4
Chocolate milkshake	1 1/2 cup	507	12.1	49.5	17.6	391	47.8
Chocolate pudding		212	4.4	29.6	3.9	161	47.1
Chocolate syrup,	2 tbsp	185	0.9	23.8	0.8	93	31.1
Cocoa	3/4 cup	203	7.1	20.4	8.6	182	55.6
Coffee, black	3/4 cup	(3)	tr	tr	tr	2	51.3
Cola	1 cup	191	0	24.6	0	96	31.2
Cookie, plain	1 3" dia.	186	1.0	18.0	5.0	120	40.0
Cookie, sugar	1 2" dia.	143	1.2	13.6	3.4	89	38.6

258

Cracker, graham	2	77	1.1	10.3	1.3	54	43.5
Cracker, saltine	5	78	1.2	9.8	1.7	60	47.7
Cupcake (with icing)	2 3/4" dia.	318	2.0	30.0	7.0	185	36.1
Danish, pastry roll	1	390	4.8	29.6	15.3	274	43.6
Donut, cake-type	1	191	1.5	16.5	6.0	125	40.6
Donut, jelly	1	382	2.5	35.0	11.0	250	40.6
French dressing	1 tbsp	65	0.1	2.8	6.2	66	63.0
Fruitcake	2 × 2 × 1/2"	138	1.0	18.0	5.0	115	51.7
Gelatin, dessert							
(sweetened)	1/2 cup	139	1.8	16.9	0	71	31.6
(unsweetened)	1/2 cup	7	1.8	tr	0	8	70.9
Highball (see Alcoholic Cocktail)							
Honey	1 tbsp	129	tr	17.0	0	65	31.2
Ice cream, vanilla	1/2 cup	190	2.7	13.7	8.3	138	45.0
Ice cream, chocolate	1/2 cup	192	2.7	14.0	8.3	140	45.2
Jell-O (see Gelatin Dessert)							
Jelly and jam	1 tbsp	74	0	12.7	0	49	41.1
Lecithin	1 tbsp	108	0	0	12	108	62.0
Mayonnaise	1 tbsp	101	0.2	0.3	11.2	101	62.0
Milkshake, chocolate	1 1/2 cup	507	12.1	49.5	17.6	391	47.8
Milkshake, vanilla	1 1/2 cup	501	12.1	48.6	17.6	387	47.9
Nuts (see Meats)							
Pastry roll, Danish	1	390	4.8	29.6	15.3	274	43.6
Peanuts (unsalted,							

Food	Serving Size	FLABs	Prote(gm)	Carbo(gm)	Fat(gm)	Cals	FLAB Index
dry roasted)	1/4 cup	181	9.4	6.8	17.9	211	72.3
Peanut butter	2 tbsp	191	8.9	5.5	15.8	200	64.9
Pie, apple	1/6 of 9"	648	3.5	60.0	17.5	403	38.6
Popcorn, plain	1 cup	9	0.8	4.6	0.3	23	100.0
Potato chips	10	126	1.1	10.0	8.0	114	56.1
Portein powder	1 oz	57	28.4	0	0	114	100.0
Pudding, chocolate	1/2 cup	212	4.4	29.6	3.9	161	47.1
Pudding, vanilla	1/2 cup	209	4.4	29.0	3.9	159	47.2
Roll, Danish pastry	1	390	4.8	29.6	15.3	274	43.6
Salad Dressing,							
Blue cheese	1 tbsp	79	1.0	1.0	8.0	80	62.8
Salad Dressing, French	1 tbsp	65	0.1	2.8	6.2	66	63.0
Salad Dressing,							
Thousand Island	1 tbsp	75	0.1	2.0	8.0	75	62.0
Soda, cola	1 cup	191	0	24.6	0	96	31.2
Soda, ginger ale	1 cup	132	0	18.0	0	70	32.9
Soft drink (see Soda)							
Sherbet, orange	1/2 cup	221	0.9	29.7	1.2	129	36.2
Syrup	1 tbsp	119	0	15.0	0	60	31.2
Sugar	1 tsp	30	0	3.7	0	15	31.0
Sugar	1 tbsp	30	0	11.2	0	45	31.0
Wine, rose	1/2 cup	95	0.1	4.3	0	87	56.8
Wine, white	1/2 cup	106	0.1	6.0	0	94	55.0

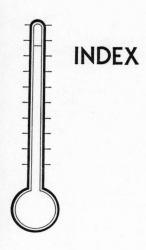

INDEX

263